D0201865

Welcome to

THE
EVERYTHING®

HEALTH GUIDES

When you're faced with a pressing health issue, your first instinct is to find out as much about it as you can. With so much conflicting information out there, where can you turn for professional, supportive advice?

Packed with the most recent, up-to-date data, THE EVERYTHING® HEALTH GUIDES help ensure that you get a good diagnosis, choose the best doctor, and find the right medical treatment. With this one comprehensive resource, you and your family members have all the information you could possibly need—at your fingertips.

THE EVERYTHING® HEALTH GUIDES are an extension of the best-selling Everything® series in the health category, which also includes *The Everything® Diabetes Book* and *The Everything® Menopause Book*. Accessible and easy to read, THE EVERYTHING® HEALTH GUIDES provide specific details and clear examples that relate to your given medical situation. If you're looking for one-stop, all-inclusive guides that allow you to understand and become more in tune with your body, this groundbreaking series is the perfect tool for you.

Visit the entire Everything® series at *www.everything.com*

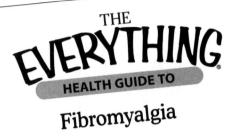

THE EVERYTHING

HEALTH GUIDE TO

Fibromyalgia

Dear Reader,

Perhaps you've been wondering if you have fibromyalgia. Or maybe you were recently diagnosed. Or perhaps you've already had it for several years and are struggling to find a way to get your symptoms under control. In any case, this book is written for you.

As a health writer and a medical doctor, we have found fibromyalgia a challenging and baffling subject. There remain so many mysteries and unanswered questions about this condition that you must have, too. What sets off the process in fibromyalgia? Why can't it be measured in simple diagnostic tests? Why are women more vulnerable than men?

Although fate may have dealt you an unlucky hand, you still have plenty of power and control over your health. You can make the choice to eat right, to exercise, and to work with your physicians. You can decide to stress less, think more positively, and explore alternative remedies. These steps alone can improve your health.

No, it's not easy to live with fibromyalgia—or any health problem, for that matter. But we hope you will take the right steps to empower yourself. Reading this book is a major step in that direction.

Sincerely,

Winnie Yu
Michael McNett, M.D.

THE
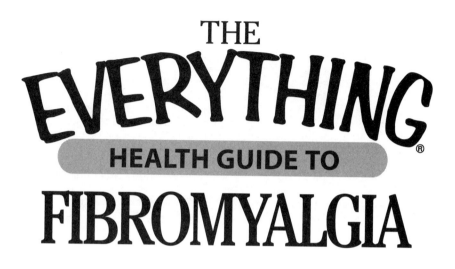

EVERYTHING
HEALTH GUIDE TO
FIBROMYALGIA

Professional advice to help you
make it through the day

Winnie Yu and Michael McNett, M.D.,
Director, Fibromyalgia Treatment
Centers of America

Adams Media
Avon, Massachusetts

Dedication
To my girls, Samantha and Stephanie—WY

• • •

Publishing Director: Gary M. Krebs
Associate Managing Editor: Laura M. Daly
Associate Copy Chief: Brett Palana-Shanahan
Acquisitions Editor: Kate Burgo
Development Editor: Jessica LaPointe
Associate Production Editor: Casey Ebert

Director of Manufacturing: Susan Beale
Associate Director of Production:
Michelle Roy Kelly
Cover Design: Paul Beatrice, Erick DaCosta,
Matt LeBlanc
Layout and Graphics: Colleen Cunningham,
Sorae Lee, Jennifer Oliveira

Copyright ©2006, F+W Publications, Inc.
All rights reserved. This book, or parts thereof, may not be reproduced
in any form without permission from the publisher; exceptions
are made for brief excerpts used in published reviews.

An Everything® Series Book.
Everything® and everything.com® are registered trademarks of F+W Publications, Inc.

Published by Adams Media, an F+W Publications Company
57 Littlefield Street, Avon, MA 02322 U.S.A.
www.adamsmedia.com

ISBN 10: 1-59337-586-7
ISBN 13: 978-1-59337-586-7
Printed in the United States of America.

J I H G F E D C B

Library of Congress Cataloging-in-Publication Data
Yu, Winnie.
The everything health guide to fibromyalgia / Winnie Yu and Michael M. McNett.
p.   cm.
Includes index.
ISBN 1-59337-586-7
1. Fibromyalgia--Popular works. I. McNett, Michael M. II. Title. III. Series.

RC927.3.Y8 2006
616.7'42--dc22
2006013591

This publication is designed to provide accurate and authoritative information with regard to the subject matter covered. It is sold with the understanding that the publisher is not engaged in rendering legal, accounting, or other professional advice. If legal advice or other expert assistance is required, the services of a competent professional person should be sought.
—From a *Declaration of Principles* jointly adopted by a Committee of the American Bar Association and a Committee of Publishers and Associations

Many of the designations used by manufacturers and sellers to distinguish their products are claimed as trademarks. Where those designations appear in this book and Adams Media was aware of a trademark claim, the designations have been printed with initial capital letters.

This book is available at quality discounts for bulk purchases.
For information, please call 1-800-289-0963.

All the examples and dialogues used in this book are fictional and have been created by the author to illustrate medical situations.

Acknowledgments

I'd like to thank my editor, Kate Burgo, who entrusted me with a topic as complex as fibromyalgia. This book also wouldn't have been possible without the support and efforts of my collaborator Michael McNett, M.D., who not only knows a great deal about fibromyalgia but has a keen eye for copy. In addition, I'd like to acknowledge Frances Jenkins, Nancy Mongato, Anita Murray, Andrea Whitaker, Elaine Burns, and Mary Delsman, who helped me better understand life with fibromyalgia. And finally, I wish to thank Jeff, Samantha, and Stephanie for simply being there.—WY

Contents

Introduction   xi

Chapter 1: Fibromyalgia Defined   1
What Is Fibromyalgia?   1
What Fibromyalgia Is Not   3
What Fibromyalgia Feels Like   4
Who Gets It?   8
Suspected Causes of Fibromyalgia   9
Conditions Associated with Fibromyalgia   12

Chapter 2: Signs and Symptoms   17
Pain: The Most Common Symptom   17
Sleep Disturbances   18
Fatigue   21
Fibro Fog and Your Brain   22
Depression   22
Irritable Bowel Syndrome (IBS)   23
Other Abdominal Issues   24
Chronic Headaches   25
Temporomandibular Joint Disorder (TMJ)   27
Raynaud's Phenomenon   28
Other Symptoms   28

Chapter 3: Fibro Imitators   31
Chronic Fatigue Immune Deficiency Syndrome (CFIDS)   31
Chronic Myofascial Pain (CMP)   34
Lupus   38
Lyme Disease   40
Hypothyroidism   43
Rheumatoid Arthritis (RA)   44
Other Conditions   46

Chapter 4: Finding the Right Doctors   49
Team Captain: You   49
Who Are the Key Players?   50
Other Specialists You Might Need   55
Finding the Best Doctor   59
What to Expect from a Good Doctor   61
The First Visit   62
Leading Your Team   63
Communicate!   65

Chapter 5: Diagnosing Fibromyalgia   **67**

The Official Word   67
A Tough Diagnosis   70
Getting to a Diagnosis   73
How You Can Help   77
Dealing with Nonbelievers   78
When You're Diagnosed   78

Chapter 6: All about Pain   **79**

What Exactly Is Pain?   79
The Nervous System   80
How Nerves Cause Pain   82
Normal Pain Versus Fibro Pain   84
What Causes Fibro Pain?   85
Body Chemicals Involved in Fibro Pain   86
The Gate Control Theory   88
Impact of Lifestyle   90

Chapter 7: The Fatigue Factor   **95**

Fibro Fatigue   95
What Makes It Worse   97
CFIDS, a Co-conspirator   98
Treating Fatigue   102
Living with Fatigue   103
Exhausting Emotions   106

Chapter 8: The Sleep Problem   **107**

What Is Sleep?   107
Fibro Sleep   108
Other Sleep Problems   110
The Insomnia Battle   113
Sleep Solutions   114
Make Sleep a Priority   116

Chapter 9: Other Fibro Troubles   **117**

The Brain   117
Headaches   120
The Eyes and Mouth   122
Tummy Troubles   124
Urinary Troubles   126
Menstrual Problems   126
Vaginal Pain   127
Problems All Over   128

Chapter 10: Medications That Can Help   **133**

Pain Relief   133
Combining Medications   139
Sleep Remedies   140
Stimulants   140
Medications for Restless Legs Syndrome (RLS)   141
Other Medications   141
Using Drugs Safely and Wisely   142
A Word on Over-the-Counter (OTC) Drugs   146
Choosing the Right One(s)   146

Chapter 11: Alternative Fibro Treatments   **149**

What Is CAM?   149
Acupuncture   150
Trigger-Point Therapy   151
Chiropractics   153
Massage   155
Reiki   157
Herbal Supplements   158
Doing the Research   163
Diet Know-How   164

Chapter 12: Living with Fibromyalgia   **167**

Adapting to Fibromyalgia   167
Listening to Your Body   170
Body Mechanics   170
Power of Posture   172
Smart Pacing   175
Let's Get Practical   177
Attitude Counts   180

Chapter 13: Staying Active   **181**

Why Exercise Matters   181
Getting Started   183
Types of Exercise   184
When Pain Strikes   189
Staying Motivated   190
Make It a Habit   191

Chapter 14: Tame the Stress Monster   **193**

The Stress Response   193
Stress and Fibromyalgia   194
Stress and Diet   196
Controlling Stress   197

Changing Your Thinking 204
Stress-Free Relationships 205

Chapter 15: Managing Difficult Emotions 207
Mourning Your Condition 207
Denial 208
Anger 208
Guilt 210
Fear 210
Loneliness 211
Coping with Emotions 212
Reaching Acceptance 218
Staying Happy 219

Chapter 16: The Mind-Body Connection 221
The Power of the Mind 221
Meditation 222
Hypnosis 223
Biofeedback 225
Guided Imagery 226
Prayer 227
Progressive Muscle Relaxation 229
Cognitive-Behavioral Therapy (CBT) 230
Other Mind-Body Techniques 230
Note the Placebo Effect 232

Chapter 17: Working and Traveling 233
Working with Fibromyalgia 233
On-the-Job Accommodations 235
Who Needs to Know? 237
Working Differently, Working Better 238
If You Become Disabled 240
Traveling with Fibro 244

Chapter 18: Fibromyalgia and Your Relationships 247
New Ways of Coping 247
Fibro and Your Marriage 248
Fibromyalgia and Children 253
Maintaining Friendships 255
Fibro Support Groups 256
Creating a Support Network 257

Chapter 19: Positive Coping 259
Take Responsibility 259

Keep Positive   262
Tap Into Your Social Network   265
Aim for Balance   267
Putting It All Together   268

Chapter 20: The Future of Fibro   269
Treatments on the Horizon   269
Revolutionary Treatments   273
The Importance of Retrograde Research   281
Toward a Better Understanding   281
Should You Assist in Research?   282
A Final Note   284

Appendix A: Organizations and Support Groups   285

Appendix B: Glossary   287

Appendix C: Further Reading   294

Index   302

Introduction

When it comes to health, knowledge is your greatest ally. Nowhere is that more true than when you're dealing with a chronic condition, especially one as complex as fibromyalgia. That's why this book is so important to people who have this condition.

If you're like most people, finding out you have fibromyalgia is only the first small step on a long journey. The diagnosis gave you a label to apply to your pain and fatigue, and it provided an explanation for why you can't seem to get a good night's rest. It helped to explain why you had no energy for long shopping sprees and why you hurt when someone hugged you too hard. But everyday living with fibromyalgia is another story, one that is often fraught with challenges, despair, and great difficulty.

Like anything, learning to live successfully with fibromyalgia takes time and practice. At first, you may bemoan the loss of your former self. You wish you still had the energy to play tennis. You wish you didn't have so many medical appointments. You wish you could still persevere in the career that you worked so hard to build. As the reality of your illness sinks in, however, you begin to realize that changes are necessary, and that the things you do can make a major impact on how well you feel. Gradually, you come to realize that taking care of your health now takes precedence over anything else you do in your life.

With that in mind, you will naturally want to learn more about fibromyalgia. That's where a book like this comes in. In this book, we give you the information, encouragement, and practical tools you need, whether you're considering an alternative treatment for your pain or figuring out what to do about your job. We also give you the basic medical knowledge you need to talk intelligently with your doctor about your condition. In addition, we give you tips and strategies that will help make your life just a little easier. And we do all this in plain English, without a lot of complicated medical-speak.

As of now, no one has all the answers to the mysteries of fibromyalgia. For instance, we still have no idea why anyone gets fibromyalgia. What is the biological mechanism or process that sets off the condition in the first place? And why does one person have a car accident and come out okay, while another one develops fibromyalgia? Those questions are best left to scientists who are working hard to improve their understanding of this perplexing condition.

What we do know now, though, is that the way you live and the choices you make can have a huge impact on how well you cope with fibromyalgia. For instance, we know that the ability to handle daily stress and difficult emotions can make a major difference in the severity of your pain. We also know that making the time and effort to both exercise and rest every day can help improve your functioning. In addition, we know that practicing good sleep hygiene—which includes treating conditions like sleep apnea—can greatly improve your sleep, which in turn will lessen your pain and fatigue. You'll find tips for doing all these things right here in this book.

No, it's not at all easy to live with fibromyalgia and its myriad symptoms and associated conditions. But the good news is that our knowledge of this condition and the treatment options we have is growing every year. In the meantime, people who have it must learn as much as they can about fibromyalgia and then work hard to make sure they are getting the best possible care.

CHAPTER 1

Fibromyalgia Defined

Most of us know the unpleasantness of a sore neck, a stiff back, or an achy muscle. And we know that awful feeling that comes with not getting a good night's rest. Most problems go away after a few days, but if you have fibromyalgia syndrome (FMS), the pain and fatigue don't go away so easily. With fibromyalgia, these symptoms persist, often for years. For some, the pain can be life altering.

What Is Fibromyalgia?

Fibromyalgia is a medical syndrome characterized by widespread pain, sleep disturbance, tender points around the body, and a host of other symptoms that range from irritable bowel syndrome to depression. It is a baffling condition and one that is hard to diagnose, commonly misdiagnosed, and difficult to treat. The cause remains a mystery, a cure elusive.

Symptoms vary widely and can change from day to day for individual patients. Most people are able to live with the disease by treating the symptoms. But in some cases, fibromyalgia can be downright debilitating. Some people have given up jobs, abandoned hobbies, and lost relationships because of fibromyalgia.

For years, people questioned whether fibromyalgia actually existed. Even today, there are skeptics who wonder whether the syndrome is real, despite the fact that millions of people suffer from these symptoms. But modern medical research has demonstrated in recent decades that fibromyalgia is very real and that people who have it have measurable differences of chemicals and substances in their bodies. These substances are associated with a hypersensitivity to pain.

Like headaches, fibromyalgia may be a symptom complex, with a number of possible causes. Just as headaches can be caused by sinus infections, migraines, muscle tension, or tumors, fibromyalgia may be associated with a neck injury, infections, stress, genetics, or compression of the upper spinal cord. Since each cause may require its own unique treatments, what works for one FMS patient may not work for others.

Fact

In the early twentieth century, doctors called fibromyalgia "fibrositis." The term comes from the Latin roots for muscle (fibro) and inflammation (itis). But over time, doctors came to realize that fibrositis was inaccurate because the condition didn't involve any inflammation. It wasn't until the late 1970s that the term "fibromyalgia" was used. The word blends the Latin term for fibrous tissue (fibro) with the Greek terms for muscle (myo) and pain (algia), and is much more accurate.

Confirming you have fibromyalgia is the first part of the struggle. Achieving relief from it is the next big challenge—and an ongoing one. These days, most people manage fibromyalgia with a host of different treatments that may include medications, diet and exercise, physical therapy, and alternative medicine. Efforts to restore sleep and alleviate depression have become routine therapies for fibromyalgia, too. Like the symptoms themselves, the treatment regimen varies, depending on the patient.

The key to living well with fibromyalgia is knowledge. Knowing as much as you can about this condition can help you minimize pain, improve sleep, and develop coping strategies that lessen the toll of fibro on every front. It will also enable you to better manage your fibromyalgia and help you continue to live a rewarding and independent life.

What Fibromyalgia Is Not

Knowing what fibromyalgia is not can be as important to your understanding of the condition as knowing what it is. Because fibromyalgia is still shrouded in mystery and the symptoms are so diverse and complex, it's easy to mistake fibromyalgia for any of several other medical conditions. But research in recent years has established certain truths about FMS that help distinguish it from other illnesses.

For starters, fibromyalgia is not arthritis, which is inflammation of the joints. Although the aches and pain of fibromyalgia may resemble those of arthritis, and the Arthritis Foundation offers information on FMS, fibro is technically not an inflammatory condition. Rheumatologists—doctors who treat arthritis, often also treat fibromyalgia. If fibromyalgia was an arthritic condition, patients could get more relief from simple anti-inflammatory medications, such as aspirin or ibuprofen. Fibromyalgia is also not usually progressive. While an occasional fibromyalgia patient may note a gradual improvement or worsening over time, FMS is not a degenerative illness and typically does not worsen with time. But that doesn't mean stress, bad weather, and too much activity won't make you feel worse on some days than others.

Fact

Too many doctors don't know how to diagnose it. Employers often don't understand it. Even loved ones have difficulties believing that the pain is real. For these reasons, the National Fibromyalgia Association in 2002 designated May 12 as Fibromyalgia Awareness Day. Each year since then, events have been held throughout the country to raise awareness of fibromyalgia.

Fibromyalgia is not psychosomatic. Skeptics have always questioned whether FMS was the product of a stressed-out lifestyle or an inability to cope. But that has slowly changed since 1990, when the American College of Rheumatology established its diagnostic criteria for fibromyalgia, and subsequent studies have proven measurable differences in people with FMS. While stress may worsen fibromyalgia, it does not appear to be the primary cause.

Fibromyalgia is not a disease. A disease is a medical condition with a specific cause or causes and distinct resulting signs and symptoms. Fibromyalgia is a syndrome, a collection of signs, symptoms, and medical problems that tend to occur together but do not appear to be related to a specific, identifiable cause. Fortunately, fibromyalgia is not life threatening. As painful as it might seem on some days, no one dies from having FMS.

What Fibromyalgia Feels Like

Diabetics may talk about blood glucose levels. Heart patients may discuss stress tests. People with osteoporosis speak of bone-density measures. But when people talk about fibromyalgia, it's often a discussion of the symptoms they're experiencing, not what's turning up in their blood work or on an X-ray. That's because medical science has not yet figured out how to measure fibro in your blood or see it on an X-ray. Doctors begin to suspect fibromyalgia when patients start describing their symptoms.

But even the signs and symptoms of fibromyalgia can vary widely from one patient to the next. That's why obtaining a diagnosis is often a struggle. Some people spend as many as five years trying to find out what is wrong. In fact, even if you're reading this book, you may still be uncertain whether what you have is fibromyalgia. Fortunately, as our understanding of the disease has grown, some symptoms have emerged as common ones. Consider the case of Dee, who wasn't properly diagnosed for twenty years:

> In her early twenties, Dee was wracked with pain and told she
> had rheumatoid arthritis. Dee lived in fear that her joints would

become deformed one day. She tried numerous RA medications, but none worked. Then, eight years ago, Dee had a car accident and learned that what she had was actually fibromyalgia. She looks back at the car accident as the event that gave her back her life and restored her hope.

You'll Feel Pain

Deep muscular aches. Sharp, shooting pains. Throbbing sensations. Those are just a few ways that fibromyalgia patients describe the chronic widespread pain that is the most common and persistent feature of fibromyalgia. Virtually all fibro patients experience some type of pain every single day. The severity of the pain can vary, depending on the weather, your stress and activity levels, and how well you've been sleeping.

Essential

For some people with fibromyalgia, everything is irritating. Ordinary lights hurt their eyes. Silk sheets irritate their skin. The hum of a car engine makes them edgy. Chalk it up to more symptoms of fibromyalgia. Some people who have FMS become hypersensitive to the sounds, smells, and sensations around them. This condition is called allodynia, which occurs when normally bearable sensations become painful ones. Interestingly, in FMS, allodynia can affect all five senses.

The pain-sensing part of a fibro patient's nervous system has been made hypersensitive. Doctors measure this by pressing on what are known as "tender points," spots scattered around your body that they use to monitor your pain sensitivity. When another person presses on these tender points—using enough force to whiten the thumbnail—you feel pain. In fibromyalgia, there are eighteen symmetrically positioned tender points that have been identified to help diagnose the disease. If more than eleven of them are tender, you qualify for a diagnosis of fibromyalgia.

You'll Feel Tired

We all have days when our energy levels are low. But in people who have fibromyalgia, the fatigue is extreme and can be physical, mental, or, most commonly, both. The fatigue in fibro is mind numbing, debilitating, and exhausting. It can make it hard for you to prepare a meal, do simple chores, or perform your job. This overwhelming weariness can make you listless and unable to exercise. In some cases, you may simply feel chronic exhaustion. Approximately 90 percent of people who have fibromyalgia experience fatigue.

You Might Feel Confused

Everyone has momentary lapses in memory, problems concentrating, and difficulties recalling the right word. But in people who have fibromyalgia, these cognitive challenges become more frequent, and you may develop what is commonly called fibro fog.

Fibro fog can result in numerous challenges. You may become absentminded, forgetful, and easily confused. Everyday objects get misplaced and turn up in strange places. Following simple directions becomes a major effort. Concentrating on a task feels like a Herculean effort. In fact, this may be a form of fatigue as well. Just as your muscles run out of energy too quickly in FMS, so can your brain cells. When they run out of energy, they don't work well anymore. It may also be a side effect of some medications used to treat fibro.

You'll Feel Sad, Maybe Anxious

People who have fibromyalgia often report feeling sad, and some may experience clinical depression. Approximately 30 percent of people with fibromyalgia are clinically depressed at any point in time. The constant pain, lack of sleep, and the struggle to pin down a diagnosis or get relief is enough to sadden even the most buoyant spirits. It is often the lack of hope and feelings of helplessness that trigger the descent into depression.

Depression can have serious ramifications, especially for people with chronic conditions that require vigilance and constant self-care. A depressed person is less likely to exercise and take her medications, and may even begin abusing drugs or alcohol. The lack of self-care can lead to a vicious cycle of despair that ultimately worsens your symptoms.

Other Problems

People who have fibromyalgia often have much more than the symptoms we've described above. Along with the pain and fatigue, you may also experience:

- Abdominal pain, bloating, diarrhea, or constipation, caused by irritable bowel syndrome, a dysfunction of the large intestine
- Painful menstrual periods
- Restless legs syndrome, an irresistible urge to move your legs
- Headaches or migraines
- Temporomandibular joint disorder
- Numbness and tingling in the extremities
- Morning stiffness

You may also experience irritable bladder; dry eyes and mouth; chronic yeast infections; Raynaud's phenomenon, an exaggerated response to the cold in the extremities; and vulvodynia, pain in the external female genitalia. We will discuss these symptoms in greater detail in Chapter 2.

Question

Why don't people believe fibro exists?
People who have it look healthy. Routine blood tests turn up nothing conclusive. X-rays and MRIs rarely reveal abnormalities in the joints or muscles. But here's the good news: Studies show that the levels of certain important chemicals are abnormal in people with fibromyalgia. In addition, scans that show brain activity levels have demonstrated that the pain centers in FMS patients are strongly hyperactive.

Who Gets It?

Though study results vary widely, the general consensus is that around 4 percent of the U.S. population has FMS. Though about 85 percent of sufferers are women, the condition does not discriminate and also affects men and children of all ages and races. More than 7 percent of women who are sixty to seventy-nine years old have FMS.

No one knows exactly what causes fibromyalgia, but certain factors do appear to increase your odds of developing FMS. Some of these risk factors are unchangeable, such as your gender and age. But you may have some control over lifestyle factors that increase your risk. The risk factors are the following:

- **Gender**—Women are about seven times more likely to get it than men.
- **Age**—Fibromyalgia is most common in women between the ages of 20 and 55.
- **Genetics**—Although scientists have not pinpointed a specific gene, the tendency to develop FMS appears to be inherited.
- **Rheumatic disease**—People who have a rheumatic illness, which involves inflammation or pain in muscles, joints, or fibrous tissue, are at greater risk of developing fibromyalgia. Rheumatic illnesses include rheumatoid arthritis, lupus, and ankylosing spondylitis.
- **Lifestyle**—People enduring major emotional or physical trauma may be at greater risk, especially if the stress is prolonged.
- **Neck injury**—Studies have shown that people who suffer a neck injury in a car accident are about thirteen times more likely to develop fibromyalgia shortly afterward than people who break their leg in one.

Several studies have suggested that being a victim of abuse increased your odds of developing a chronic pain condition, such as fibromyalgia. In 2005, a study published in the *Journal of Clinical*

Rheumatology reported that patients with rheumatic diseases, including fibro, were more likely to have had a history of verbal, physical, and sexual abuse. Among patients with fibromyalgia, more than 70 percent said they had been victims of abuse.

Suspected Causes of Fibromyalgia

As of now, no one knows exactly what sets off the constellation of symptoms we know as fibromyalgia. It's quite possible that there are multiple triggers. It's also possible that the cause is different for different people, just as the symptoms are. But there is certainly no shortage of theories as to what the culprit might be.

Central Nervous System Defect

The pain associated with fibromyalgia is most likely the result of an abnormality in your central nervous system (CNS), which is made up of your brain and spine. The CNS processes and coordinates the nerve signals it receives from the peripheral nervous system, including those that alert you to pain. Pain is a normal reaction to a potentially harmful external stimulus and acts as your body's internal alarm system.

In people who have fibro, there appears to be a defect in the CNS sensory processing that alerts us to pain. For starters, fibro patients tend to have more nerves involved in transmitting pain. In addition, the internal "computers" that process pain are overactive. As a result, pain signals are intensified. The supercharged signals in turn create more nerve connections in your spine that perpetuate the cycle of pain.

Physical Trauma or Injury

Many experts believe that the pain and fatigue of fibromyalgia may result from certain types of physical trauma. Neck injuries, in particular, seem to bring on the symptoms of fibro. So if someone is genetically predisposed to getting fibromyalgia, as experts suspect, an accident or injury could be the environmental trigger that sets off the condition.

Illness or Infection

In some people, the onset of fibromyalgia is preceded by an illness, raising the prospect that FMS is brought on by infection. Possible culprits include Lyme disease, hepatitis, and the Epstein-Barr virus, which causes mononucleosis. Illness or infection as a cause, however, fails to explain the cases that seem to appear from out of nowhere with no prior illness.

Emotional Stress

Many people with fibromyalgia note that they were going through periods of severe emotional stress around the time their symptoms started. Divorce, the death of a loved one, or professional/financial hardships all can increase the risk of developing fibromyalgia. It is rare, however, for FMS to develop without other factors also being present.

Question

Is there a link between the Gulf War and fibromyalgia?
Scientists aren't sure, but upon returning from the war in 1991, many veterans complained of excessive fatigue and joint pain. More recently, a study by the Department of Veteran Affairs published in 2005 in the *Annals of Internal Medicine* found that Gulf War veterans were 66 percent more likely to have fibro than those who had not been deployed.

Hormonal and Chemical Disturbances

Some experts believe that fibromyalgia is precipitated by hormonal changes and chemical disturbances. Hormones are chemicals in the body that regulate specific activities of different organs. Among the hormones that are altered or affected in people with fibro are those described in the following sections.

Substance P

Substance P is a chemical that increases your nerves' sensitivity to pain. In people with FMS, the amount of substance P found in spinal fluid is three times the normal amount of that in healthy people.

Serotonin

Serotonin is a neurotransmitter involved in regulating pain and mood. It also facilitates sound sleep. In people with fibromyalgia, serotonin levels are commonly lower than normal.

HPA Axis Hormones

The hypothalamic-pituitary-adrenal (HPA) axis is responsible for the release of hormones that help you cope with stress. In people who have fibro, there may be an imbalance of hormones in the HPA axis, which hinders the body's fight-or-flight response and renders it less effective.

Growth Hormones

Growth hormones are secreted during the deepest stages of sleep and play a role in helping the body rebuild itself. People who have FMS generally have lower levels of growth hormones. Some studies have shown that correcting these levels by giving patients growth hormone may significantly reduce FMS symptoms.

Sleep Disturbance

It's hard to say whether sleep difficulties cause fibromyalgia, result from it, or both. But some people believe that sleep difficulties are at the root of this condition. Studies have found that even healthy people who had fragmented stage 4 sleep, the deepest stage of sleep, were susceptible to the aches and pains seen in fibromyalgia. It is during this critical stage of sleep that our bodies restore themselves and secrete important immune-boosting substances and growth hormone.

Conditions Associated with Fibromyalgia

It's common to have fibromyalgia at the same time you have another illness. In fact, certain medical conditions may predispose you to developing FMS. These coexisting conditions can make diagnosis more difficult because the symptoms may overlap. It often takes the efforts of a skilled physician to determine whether you have two or more distinct medical conditions. The following sections describe some conditions that often occur at the same time you have fibromyalgia.

Chronic Fatigue Immune Deficiency Syndrome (CFIDS)

People who have chronic fatigue immune deficiency syndrome (CFIDS) experience extreme, bone-crushing fatigue that persists for months and does not respond to rest. More specifically, CFIDS is characterized by chronic fatigue that has lasted six months or more. You may also have muscle pain, joint pain, impaired memory, headaches, sore throat, and fever. Usually, blood tests are normal and done to rule out other conditions rather than pin down a diagnosis of CFIDS.

Fact

Back in the mid-1980s, some researchers found that people who had symptoms of CFIDS had more evidence of infection by the Epstein-Barr virus than normal. The Epstein-Barr virus causes mononucleosis, and, in fact, many people suspected of having CFIDS did indeed have mono a few years before. Researchers have since learned that EBV is not proof of CFIDS. Even healthy people can demonstrate high levels of antibodies against EBV, while some people with CFIDS may not.

Some experts believe that CFIDS is the same thing as fibromyalgia. But people who have CFIDS don't usually have tender points, and evidence suggests that CFIDS is usually triggered by a virus. The possibility of a viral link to FMS remains controversial. Still, many people who have fibromyalgia also have CFIDS.

Chronic Myofascial Pain

Chronic myofascial pain (CMP) is a medical term for persistent muscle pain associated with the presence of small spastic knots in the muscles. Pressing on these knots reproduces the pain, which sometimes occurs at quite a distance from the site of the knot itself.

CMP may involve a single muscle or a muscle group. In the aftermath of trauma—be it a car accident, an injury, or another major stressor—chemical changes occur in the nerve endings, making them secrete large amounts of the chemicals that cause muscles to contract. The high local concentration of these chemicals causes a spastic knot that restricts blood flow, causing more spasm, and a vicious cycle that allows the trigger point to persist. In addition, the low blood flow to the area activates pain fibers, resulting in a pain most commonly described as resembling a toothache.

It is very common for people to have both fibromyalgia and CMP. After all, the conditions share a great deal in common. But the two conditions remain separate and distinct. The primary difference is that fibro patients have pain because their nerves are hypersensitive, while myofascial patients have pain because their muscles are in spasm. The key is to determine whether you have one or the other syndrome, or possibly both.

Lupus

Systemic lupus erythematosus (SLE) is an autoimmune disorder that occurs when the body's immune system attacks the chromosomes of its own cells. The result is a chronic inflammatory condition that can cause a red rash, painful joints, a persistent fever, and extreme fatigue. In some cases, SLE can affect vital organs such as the kidneys or brain, and it may even be fatal. Another kind of lupus, discoid lupus, is less severe and confined to the skin.

More than 90 percent of people with SLE experience joint and/or muscle pain at some time during their illness. The main cause of pain in SLE is inflammation of the tissues due to the autoimmune attack. But sometimes the pain may be the result of another condition such as fibromyalgia. Among people who have lupus, approximately 10 to 40 percent will also eventually develop fibromyalgia.

Rheumatoid Arthritis

Like lupus, rheumatoid arthritis is an autoimmune disease. In this case, the body's immune system mistakenly attacks the membrane lining the joints, resulting in a decrease in your range of motion, pain, stiffness, swelling, and a feeling of warmth in the affected area.

It's easy to confuse the symptoms of RA with those of fibromyalgia. Both cause morning stiffness, pain, and achiness. But RA causes inflammation in the joints, while fibromyalgia does not. Like lupus, approximately 10 to 40 percent of people who have RA will develop fibromyalgia, too.

Lyme Disease

Lyme disease is caused by the *Borrelia burgdorferi* bacterium, which is transmitted by deer ticks. When an infected tick bites a human or animal, it can pass along the bacterium, which then travels into the bloodstream and causes a number of symptoms, some of which can be quite severe.

 Alert

To prevent Lyme disease, steer clear of tick-infested areas, especially during the spring and summer. When outside, wear long sleeves and pants and tuck pants into socks or boot tops. Use insect repellent that contains DEET or permethrin, a chemical that kills ticks on contact. Check frequently for deer ticks, and, if you find one, call your doctor for instructions on how to remove it.

Usually, Lyme disease begins with a circular rash that resembles a bull's eye around the site of the bite and evolves into a flu-like illness.

Caught early, the disease can be treated with a regimen of antibiotics. In later stages, it can cause neurological problems, arthritis, and numbness. In some people, having Lyme disease triggers the onset of fibromyalgia. It has been found that not even prompt treatment with antibiotics helps alleviate the symptoms of FMS.

Other Concurrent Illnesses

Knowing you have fibromyalgia may not bring about the relief you want from bothersome symptoms. That's why it's important to determine whether you have other medical conditions, too. Those cited in preceding sections are the main ones that often coexist with FMS, but they are by no means the only conditions. Other diseases that may occur at the same time as fibromyalgia include these:

- Osteoarthritis
- Hypothyroidism
- Clinical depression
- Irritable bowel syndrome
- Multiple sclerosis
- Post-traumatic stress syndrome
- Temporomandibular joint disorder
- Chronic yeast infections
- Vulvodynia

If you suspect you have any of these other conditions, talk to your doctor. Treating these conditions can sometimes help alleviate symptoms associated with fibromyalgia.

CHAPTER 2

Signs and Symptoms

Sure, you've hurt before. You've been tired and had trouble sleeping before, too. But now it feels as if the pain has intensified tenfold, and your fatigue has become unbearable. You can no longer blame your symptoms on advancing age or a hectic lifestyle. You're starting to suspect—or even know—that you have fibromyalgia. In this chapter, we'll help you zero in on what you might be experiencing.

Pain: The Most Common Symptom

Everyone who has fibromyalgia suffers pain of some sort. Although widespread pain is hardly exclusive to fibromyalgia, it is the cornerstone for diagnosing people with FMS. Some people might feel it in their hips. Others might experience it in their shoulders. Still others might simply hurt all over. The type of pain varies, too. It might be deep muscular aches or knife-like stabs of sharp pain. It could be a dull, throbbing sensation or a burning feeling. In any case, the pain of fibromyalgia is chronic, which means that while it may improve or even go away completely, it always comes back.

Often, the pain is worse when you first wake up. You may also feel stiff after prolonged periods of sitting. From one day to the next, the pain may travel from one part of your body to another. Stress, weather, and anxiety can make the aches worse on some days than others. Before you can be diagnosed with fibromyalgia, the pain must have been present for at least three months.

Fact

More than half of all Americans suffer from chronic and recurrent pain, according to a 2005 poll of 1,204 adults by ABC News, *USA Today*, and the Stanford University Medical Center. Nineteen percent said their pain was chronic, and 34 percent said it was recurrent. The most painful site? Twenty-five percent of the respondents reported having back pain.

Where It Hurts

Any part of your body is susceptible to pain when you have fibromyalgia. Pain is considered widespread if it occurs in all four quadrants of the body, meaning you hurt on both the left and right sides of your body and that the aches are both above and below the waist.

Often the pain shifts. It might be in your shoulders one day, the hips the next. On the third day, you might have a pounding headache. Some people say fibro pain resembles the aches you commonly experience with the flu.

The Tender Points

The way doctors diagnose fibromyalgia is by checking for tenderness at eighteen specific sites on your body. A doctor looking for tender points will do palpations, a technique that involves pressing down on a suspected site until his nail whitens. Before you can be diagnosed with FMS, at least eleven of these spots must be painful.

Sleep Disturbances

Like diet and exercise, a good night's rest is essential to our health. It restores, rejuvenates, and recharges our bodies so that we can function safely and effectively. But in people who have FMS, sound sleep is rare. It's unclear whether poor sleep is a cause of fibromyalgia or a result of it. In any case, estimates show that 60 to 90 percent of people who have fibromyalgia do not sleep well. Sleep can be difficult for several reasons.

Alpha-EEG Anomaly

To get restful sleep, a person must get enough of each of the five stages of sleep every night. The five stages are stage one (dozing), stage two (moderate), stage three (deep), stage four (very deep), and REM (dream) sleep stages. (Chapter 8 discusses sleep stages in greater detail.) It is during stages three and four (known as the delta stages) that the muscles are best able to repair the wear and tear that occurs during the day. It is also then that we release the greatest amount of growth hormone, a substance vital to metabolism, restorative sleep, and muscle repair and growth.

In people who have fibromyalgia, sleep during the deeper delta stages is disrupted by alpha brain waves, which normally occur when you're awake but relaxed, causing a condition known as alpha-EEG anomaly, or alpha-delta intrusion. The intrusion of alpha brain waves jolts you back to a shallower level of sleep and cheats you of the restorative sleep your body needs. The next day, you awaken feeling tired and unrefreshed, even if you've slept through the night.

Stimulation

Trying to sleep with pain is like trying to sleep during a rock concert. Both are stimulating the brain. The only difference is that during a rock concert, the stimulation is coming from your ears, while with pain the stimulation is coming from your body. A stimulated brain has trouble relaxing and slipping into the deep sleep stages. As a result, sleep quality becomes poor, and you awaken wondering if you actually slept at all.

Insomnia

Almost everyone has the occasional night when she can't fall asleep or awakens in the wee hours of dawn. Both of these situations are forms of insomnia. According to a poll by the National Sleep

Foundation, 58 percent of all U.S. adults experience insomnia a few nights a week or more.

Insomnia can present itself in different ways. If you have trouble falling asleep, you have sleep onset insomnia. If you constantly awaken in the middle of the night, you are said to have maintenance insomnia. Those who wake up too early in the morning and can't get back to sleep have early A.M. insomnia.

Restless Legs Syndrome (RLS)

Approximately 20 to 40 percent of people with FMS suffer from a neurological condition called restless legs syndrome (RLS). The condition is quite common, and experts estimate that 8 percent of all adults in the U.S. experience RLS.

The condition typically occurs at night and makes your legs feel twitchy, uneasy, and tingly, which causes an overwhelming urge to move the legs. The only way to get relief from these uncomfortable sensations is to get up and move.

Periodic Leg Movements During Sleep (PLMS)

About 80 percent of people with RLS also have periodic leg movements during sleep. PLMS is characterized by purposeless maneuvers of the legs and feet. The involuntary motion is sometimes strong enough to hurt someone sleeping beside you. The movements, which may occur as often as every half a second, can be small and imperceptible or wild and flailing. Rarely, the movement may involve the arms. In any case, the involuntary nighttime motions inhibit sound sleep and leave its sufferers (and their partners!) exhausted.

Sleep Apnea

People who have sleep apnea actually stop breathing for ten to thirty seconds at a time while they are asleep. These brief spells can occur as many as 400 times a night. The breathing disruptions may awaken you and prevent you from getting a good night's rest. For some people, sleep apnea can be fatal.

Most people with sleep apnea have obstructive apnea, which means something is blocking the windpipe, or trachea, that brings air into the body. Efforts to breathe are blocked by the tongue, tonsils, or uvula, the little piece of flesh that hangs in the back of your throat. Excess fatty tissue in the throat or even relaxed throat muscles can cause obstructive sleep apnea, too. Sleep apnea is more common in men with fibromyalgia than women.

Alert

If you snore on a regular basis or suffer from excessive sleepiness during the day, you may have sleep apnea. Other symptoms include morning headaches, poor memory and concentration, and waking up gasping or choking for air. Men may experience impotence. If you suspect you have it, ask your doctor for a sleep study.

Fatigue

In many FMS patients, fatigue is as big a life-destroyer as pain. There are many possible causes of fatigue. Some people feel it's due to abnormal nervous system responses. Others blame low levels of growth hormone. Still others think it's caused by inhibition of the chemical reactions that burn sugar to create energy. Whatever the cause, fatigue can be debilitating. Among fibro patients who go on disability, most cite fatigue as the primary reason.

One treatable factor that worsens fatigue is poor sleep. Even the healthiest people will experience fatigue without a good night's rest. But it can also be brought on by stress, anxiety, and a busy schedule. In people with FMS, the situation is made worse by unrelenting pain and the stress of having a chronic condition. Many patients find, however, that if their sleep is improved with medications, fatigue is reduced.

Muscular fatigue is also a major problem in FMS sufferers. Many people with fibro note that they are physically incapable of activities that used to be commonplace for them, such as walking through a grocery store, picking up their child, or doing routine job activities like typing. It's easy to imagine how devastating this could be for someone living alone, or how many problems it could cause for a FMS patient's family. In some people, muscular fatigue may get so bad that they are confined to a wheelchair.

Fibro Fog and Your Brain

People who have fibromyalgia may experience difficulties in their ability to think, analyze, and remember things. These problems are commonly referred to as fibro fog. For some people, these cognitive challenges are the most frustrating symptoms of all. With fibro fog, you have difficulty remembering familiar names, you misplace every-day objects, and you struggle to focus and concentrate. You may become easily confused and disoriented. Doing your job, perform-ing daily tasks, and following simple directions can become monu-mental challenges in the grip of fibro fog.

Poor sleep contributes to fibro fog. Experts suspect that people with fibromyalgia may have low brain metabolism, possibly as a result of getting less oxygen into their brains. Other possible causes include depression, a malfunction in the central nervous system, and certain medications, including some used to treat fibromyalgia.

Depression

Like any chronic illness, fibromyalgia can take a toll on your mood. The unrelenting pain, lack of sleep, and persistent fatigue can dampen even the most lighthearted spirits. As a result, you may start to feel hopeless and sad, which can spiral into a case of full-blown depression.

We all have days when we're feeling down, but depression is much more than that. People who have depression feel a persistent sadness or emptiness, and they often feel hopeless and pessimistic about life. They may also experience feelings of guilt, worthlessness, or helplessness. Hobbies and activities that they once pursued with zeal are suddenly no longer enjoyable.

In people who have fibromyalgia, depression can be hazardous. Being depressed can make it harder for you to take care of yourself, to eat well and exercise, and to follow your doctor's instructions. It can make you negligent about your health. If severe enough, it may result in suicidal thoughts or actions. Depression should never be taken lightly and should be brought to the attention of a health-care professional.

Fact

According to the National Institutes of Mental Health, suicide is the eleventh leading cause of death in the United States. Signs of suicidal thoughts include discussions of suicide, statements of hopelessness, and a preoccupation with death. Once someone decides to commit suicide, the person may seem happier or calmer for no apparent reason. Seek professional help if you or someone you love displays these behaviors.

Irritable Bowel Syndrome (IBS)

Irritable bowel syndrome (IBS) is a chronic gastrointestinal condition characterized by cramps, abdominal pain, bloating, constipation, and diarrhea. No one knows exactly what causes IBS, but we do know it involves a malfunction of the large intestine. Nerves and muscles in the large intestine may contract too much or be overly sensitive to certain stimuli such as foods or stress. As a result, stool may pass too quickly or slowly through the intestines, resulting in diarrhea or constipation.

For sufferers, IBS can be extremely disruptive. The unpredictability and discomfort of the symptoms can make it hard for you to travel, do your job, or socialize with friends. But as annoying as it is, the condition does not cause permanent damage to the intestines and does not lead to serious diseases such as cancer.

As many as 20 percent of all adults in the United States suffer from IBS, and most of them are women. The condition afflicts approximately 70 percent of people with fibromyalgia. If you have these symptoms, however, don't just assume you have IBS. These can also be symptoms of other intestinal diseases. Be sure to get checked out by an intestinal specialist, known as a gastroenterologist.

Essential

Younger people who suffer from persistent diarrhea should be checked for inflammatory bowel disease, also known as Crohn's disease. Crohn's is a chronic autoimmune condition, in which the body attacks its gastrointestinal tract. Symptoms typically come and go, and the disease is treated with a combination of medications and dietary modifications.

Other Abdominal Issues

Aside from irritable bowel syndrome, fibro sufferers often present other disorders that affect the lower abdominal and pelvic areas.

Interstitial Cystitis

People who have fibromyalgia are more likely to have interstitial cystitis, a chronic hyperactivity of the bladder that can cause discomfort and pain in the bladder and surrounding pelvic region. If you have interstitial cystitis, you may experience an increased need to urinate, and it may feel urgent. In severe cases, some people urinate as many as sixty times a day. Interstitial cystitis can also cause pain in the pelvic region, especially during sexual intercourse and/or menstruation.

Vulvodynia

Vulvodynia is chronic pain or discomfort of the vulva, or external female genitalia. Women may experience burning, stinging, irritation, or rawness, but there is no infection or skin disease. The pain may be constant or intermittent.

Vulvodynia can make it hard for women to engage in sexual activity. It can also interfere with their daily functioning and may cause depression. Again, myofascial trigger points that are a part of chronic myofascial pain are often associated with vulvodynia.

Painful Periods and PMS

It's not unusual for healthy women to battle monthly cramps and pain during their periods. And in the days leading up to their periods, they may suffer from premenstrual syndrome, a constellation of symptoms that includes moodiness, bloating, and water retention. In women with fibromyalgia, your monthly period may become even more painful. You may experience more cramps, irregular blood flow, blood clots, or larger than normal blood flow. In addition, your PMS symptoms may become intensified.

Chronic Headaches

According to the American Council on Headache Education, 90 percent of men and 95 percent of women experienced a headache in the past year.

People who have fibromyalgia may be more vulnerable to headaches than the average person. Approximately 50 percent of people with fibromyalgia suffer from recurrent migraine or tension headaches. Chronic headaches of any kind can be disruptive and interfere with daily activities.

Migraine Headaches

Nearly 30 million people in the United States suffer from migraine headaches, the vast majority of them women. Migraine headaches are a specific type of headache, characterized by intense pain that often occurs on one side of the head and that gets worse with ordinary activities. In the early and later phases of a migraine attack, you may experience muscle tenderness, fatigue, and mood changes. You may also feel nauseous and even vomit. The severity of a migraine and what triggers it varies a great deal. Migraines can last four to seventy-two hours or more.

Some migraine attacks may be accompanied by what experts call an aura, which is an abnormal sensory experience. During an aura, you may see zigzag lines, shimmering lights, or bright flashes of lights. An aura may also be accompanied by numbness and tingling in the arm, and you may need to lie down in a dark place until it passes.

Thirteen million U.S. women suffer from menstrual migraines, which can last longer and recur more often than regular migraine headaches. Some women have pure menstrual migraines that occur during their period. Others suffer from menstrual-related migraines, which can occur any time of the month. No one knows what causes menstrual migraines, but experts suspect that the drop in estrogen levels during menstruation may be the cause. Birth control pills are also associated with menstrual migraines because they cause changes in estrogen levels.

Tension Headaches

Tension headaches, which are more common than migraines, afflict approximately 78 percent of all adults. They are generally the result of tight muscles in the neck or shoulders and are commonly associated with myofascial trigger points.

In the throes of a tension headache, you might feel as if you have a band tightening around your neck or head. You may feel a pressing sensation on both sides of the head, and it may involve the temples, the back of the head, and/or the neck. Routine activities don't worsen the pain, and you are not sensitive to light or noise.

Numerous factors can trigger a headache. Certain foods, odors, your period, and the weather can all set off the pain. Stress, depression, anxiety, disappointment, and frustration also can cause headaches. Too much time in front of a computer, sleeping in an awkward position, and overuse of caffeine can all trigger a headache. To pinpoint the cause of your pain, keep a headache diary and record the circumstances that surrounded the pain, including foods you ate, your mood, how well you slept the night before, and even the weather. After a while, you should see a pattern.

Alert

It's tempting to reach for an over-the-counter pain reliever when your head is pounding. But overusing these remedies can cause a rebound effect that only triggers more headaches. The rebound effect is most common in people who are susceptible to headaches and who take pain relievers more than two days a week for weeks at a time. So try to minimize your use of these analgesics if at all possible.

Temporomandibular Joint Disorder (TMJ)

Every time you talk, chew, yawn, or laugh, you exercise your temporomandibular joint. This critical joint connects the upper jaw to the lower jaw. People who have temporomandibular joint disorder (TMJ) may experience stiffness, headaches, ear pain, or grinding and clicking noises in their jaw. In some cases, the jaws may even lock. About half of TMJ cases are caused by irritation of the joint itself. The other half is due to myofascial pain in the surrounding muscles.

TMJ affects more than 10 million people in the United States, most of them women in their childbearing years. Research suggests that hormones may be the culprit. A study done in 1997 by researchers at the University of Washington in Seattle found that women on hormone replacement were more than 70 percent more likely to seek treatment for TMJ than those not on hormone therapy. Similarly, women who take oral contraceptives were 20 percent more likely to have TMJ than those who did not.

TMJ typically occurs when you grind and clench your teeth at night, a condition called bruxism. The grinding and clenching is believed to the result of daytime stress.

Raynaud's Phenomenon

Blood vessels are supposed to constrict when they're exposed to cold temperatures; that's the body's way of preserving heat. But in people who have Raynaud's, the blood vessels undergo vasospasms that reduce circulation to the extremities, causing fingers, toes, and even the tips of your nose or ears to turn white. When they recover, the extremities turn red and tingle.

Being outdoors in frigid weather, however, isn't the only thing that can set off an attack. Stress, cigarette smoking, and even a stroll through the freezer section of a supermarket can trigger an attack. Raynaud's may be a primary condition that exists on its own, or it can be a secondary condition in people who have fibromyalgia, lupus, or scleroderma.

If you do experience Raynaud's, try to warm up the affected body parts quickly. Persistent severe Raynaud's can cause a reduction in blood flow severe enough to injure or kill the involved tissues.

Other Symptoms

People who have fibromyalgia are vulnerable to a host of medical conditions. We've described some of the more common, but they are by no means the only ones. In addition, you may experience some other symptoms:

- Dry eyes and mouth
- Numbness or tingling
- Chronic yeast infections
- Sensitive skin and rashes
- Anxiety

Not everyone will experience all these symptoms. Some people may experience only the pain and fatigue, while others may be hit with several at once. Other people may not have these symptoms now but may develop them years later.

No matter what the signs or symptoms, you should always discuss them with your doctor. It's important to rule out other, possibly serious conditions that could cause these symptoms. Fibromyalgia patients get sick just as other people do who don't have FMS. And many other illnesses can cause symptoms that overlap with FMS. Any time you develop a new condition or symptom, resist the temptation to just write it off as fibro. See your doctor and get checked out.

Fibro Imitators

Sometimes, knowing what something isn't can be as important as knowing what it is. That's true with fibromyalgia. The symptoms of FMS overlap with so many other maladies that you could be misdiagnosed several times before learning you have fibromyalgia. Getting a better understanding of these other conditions can help you figure out whether you actually have fibromyalgia or something else. This chapter examines six of the most common imitators.

Chronic Fatigue Immune Deficiency Syndrome (CFIDS)

Fatigue has become a part of the human condition. But chronic fatigue and immune deficiency syndrome (CFIDS), also called chronic fatigue syndrome (CFS), is more insidious than normal tiredness. With CFIDS, the fatigue is strong, persistent, and debilitating, typically making you too weak to perform everyday tasks. Often, you're tired even when you have little to do or after a good night's rest. Many people say that the fatigue of CFIDS is similar to the fatigue of the flu.

According to estimates by the U.S. Centers for Disease Control and Prevention, approximately 500,000 Americans suffer from CFIDS. Most people with CFIDS are women. In the 1980s, CFIDS was called the "yuppie flu" because most sufferers were well-educated, middle-to-upper-class women in their thirties and forties. But now we know that CFIDS can afflict anyone of any age, and that people of any race or socioeconomic level can be affected.

Today, the cause of CFIDS remains a mystery, though research suggests that a chronic, low-grade viral infection may be present. Usually, a diagnosis is made only after other medical conditions are ruled out. But like fibromyalgia, CFIDS can coexist with other disorders such as depression. It can also resemble other illnesses, such as hypothyroidism.

Fact

A study done in England and published in the *British Medical Journal* found that a lack of exercise in childhood may be linked to a greater risk for developing CFIDS in adulthood. The study looked at 16,567 babies born in April of 1970 and followed them until they were thirty years old.

Symptoms and Diagnosis

Getting a diagnosis of CFIDS can be difficult. There are no laboratory tests or clinical signs that characterize the condition, so doctors must rely on patient reports of specific symptoms. To make matters more challenging, some people are still skeptical that the condition even exists.

But a scientific panel of experts did come up with a set of criteria for CFIDS, which was first published in the *Annals of Internal Medicine* in March 1988 and revised in the same journal in December 1994. According to those criteria, you may be diagnosed with CFIDS if you have severe chronic fatigue that has lasted longer than six months without the presence of any other medical conditions. At the same time, you must have at least four or more of the following symptoms:

- Substantial impairment in short-term memory or concentration
- Sore throat
- Tender lymph nodes
- Muscle pain

- Joint pain in several joints without swelling or redness
- Headaches that seem different in severity, type, and pattern than those you've experienced in the past
- Unrefreshing sleep
- A feeling of malaise after exertion, lasting more than twenty-four hours

Other symptoms of CFIDS include fever, abdominal cramps, allergies, weight loss, rapid pulse, chest pain, night sweats, rash, and chest pain.

But your doctor won't diagnose you with CFIDS if you have another documented illness that can cause chronic fatigue, such as cancer or hepatitis. Interestingly, fibromyalgia was specifically excluded from this rule, so it is possible to have both CFIDS and FMS.

Treating CFIDS

Unfortunately, there is no treatment for CFIDS at the current time. But certain lifestyle strategies can lessen the symptoms. Eating a balanced diet, getting enough sleep, and exercising regularly can all help. Studies show that even moderate amounts of exercise can reduce the symptoms in 75 percent of people with CFIDS. Strategies to minimize stress can help, too. Avoid doing too much, and practice strategies for managing stress, such as meditation or tai chi.

Some people find relief from CFIDS by taking antidepressants. Low-dose tricyclic antidepressants such as Elavil or selective serotonin reuptake inhibitors (SSRIs) such as Prozac have been shown to provide relief by improving the quality of sleep and decreasing the fatigue, not necessarily by relieving depression.

How CFIDS Differs from FMS

Even doctors can't always separate CFIDS from FMS. Patients with CFIDS often experience some pain, while those with FMS are frequently fatigued. As a result, a person diagnosed with fibromyalgia by one doctor may be told he has CFIDS by another, which can be very confusing.

But subtle differences do exist. Fibromyalgia is often linked to an injury or trauma. CFIDS typically starts off like flu. People who have CFIDS typically don't have tender points. And in research, CFIDS sufferers are less likely to have abnormal levels of substance P or serotonin the way fibro sufferers do.

Chronic Myofascial Pain (CMP)

People who have fibromyalgia often have symptoms of chronic myofascial pain (CMP) too. But CMP, like CFIDS, is a syndrome unto itself. Experts believe that CMP originates with a muscle lesion or strain on a particular muscle, ligament, or tendon, which in turn creates a small spastic knot called a trigger point. Trigger points cause local pain and often send pain to other parts of the body—called referred pain—sometimes quite a ways from the location of the trigger point. CMP may also come on as a result of fatigue, repetitive motion, a medical condition, or lack of activity.

To better understand CMP, consider the word myofascial. "Myo" means muscle and "fascia" means connective tissue. So myofascial pain stems from problems in muscles and connective tissue. This makes it different from FMS, which is the result of oversensitivity in the parts of your nervous system responsible for sensing and processing pain.

It appears that irritation or damage to muscles can, in some cases, cause a change in the nerves responsible for telling the muscle to contract. As a result, instead of just telling the muscle to work when you want it to, the nerve starts constantly releasing chemicals that activate the muscle. This causes that local area of muscle to go into a tight, spastic knot that actually reduces blood flow. As a result of the decrease in blood flow, the area doesn't get the oxygen it needs, and lactic acid (among other things) starts to build up. This activates nerves in the area, causing pain.

The trigger point causes pain when you try to move, and you lose range of motion. As you become increasingly resistant to moving, other muscles are summoned to compensate for the weakness. Once these other muscles are overworked, they too become vulnerable to the development of trigger points. The resulting pain is typically steady, dull, deep, and can be anything from mild to excruciating.

Alert

Holding a muscle in an awkward position can lead to the development of a trigger point. Sitting in a chair with poor back support, using your shoulder to hold a phone to your ear, and prolonged bending over a desk can all create trigger points. Other perpetuating factors include emotional stress, sports injuries, and poor posture.

Symptoms and Diagnosis

People who have CMP complain about regional pain that is persistent and restricts motion. Often, the neck, shoulder, low back, and pelvic muscles are affected. You may experience tension headaches, tinnitus (a ringing of the ears), temporomandibular joint disorder, joint pain, vision problems, and torticollis (wry neck). CMP does not cause systemic problems such as joint swelling.

The key to diagnosing CMP is identifying trigger points in muscles that reproduce pain when pressed. There are actually four different kinds of trigger points, which can all be felt by palpation. Palpation is the application of pressure—usually by the diagnosing physician—on a suspected trigger point, which causes tremendous pain.

Active Trigger Points

Active trigger points spontaneously hurt, are extremely sensitive to touch, and can cause both local and referred pain. When pressed, active trigger points can sometimes produce severe pain.

Latent Trigger Points

Latent trigger points don't hurt unless someone is pressing on them. But they still cause muscle tension, restrict movement, and weaken the muscle. They can become active due to lack of exercise, injury, infection, or stress.

Secondary Trigger Points

When a muscle gets overused as the result of a trigger point elsewhere, a secondary trigger point can develop. Secondary trigger points result from muscle compensation and become highly irritable.

Satellite Trigger Points

Satellite trigger points are located inside an inactive muscle that is located in the referred pain area of an active trigger point. These trigger points are also quite irritable.

At this time, there are no lab tests or imaging studies that can diagnose CMP. Diagnosis is based on patient's self-reported pain and the ability to reproduce that pain by pressing on trigger points.

Essential

The Alexander Technique is a method that reeducates your body's movements. The method helps you ditch old habits of moving that cause discomfort and pain and helps you adopt new ways to move that are more fluid and effortless. Devotees say it can help avoid repetitive stress injuries, cure a stiff neck, and even enhance your voice.

Treating CMP

Eliminating the pain of CMP usually requires a combination of passive and active forms of physical therapy. The most common treatment is to press on the trigger point while the muscle is being stretched. This pressure should be right between "good" hurt and "bad" hurt. Some patients are given the stretch-and-spray treatment, which involves spraying the affected muscle with a coolant, then slowly stretching it. Others may undergo complementary therapies, such as massage, acupuncture, and the application of heat and cold.

In some cases, patients are given trigger-point injections of different substances including an anesthesia such as lidocaine or botulinum toxin A. Sometimes a corticosteroid is added to the treatment. But corticosteroids add little benefit and significantly increase the risk of side effects. Treatment may also involve medications for pain and sleep and/or muscle relaxants.

How CMP Differs from FMS

If you're unfortunate enough to have both conditions you may not be able to distinguish one from the other. Both conditions cause sleep disturbances and depression. And although you can have CMP and FMS at the same time, the two conditions are actually quite different.

For instance, CMP is the result of trigger points, which may occur anywhere on the body, alone or in multiple locations. Trigger points also cause referred pain, so that a trigger point on the upper back may cause pain to resonate into the lower arm.

Alert

People who have just FMS can manage some slow and gentle stretches, but if you suspect you have CMP, beware of physical therapy. Done incorrectly, it can worsen your pain. So look for a certified myofascial therapist with the skill it takes to do physical therapy on myofascial pain. Keep in mind that a myofascial therapist doesn't have to be a physical therapist to be good.

People with FMS but not CMP do not suffer from restricted motion and will not feel the hard lumps or tight, ropy bands that are characteristic of trigger points in CMP. In addition, FMS does not cause referred pain. The pain of pure FMS tends to move around without obvious reasons, and it is not reproduced by pressure on a specific site. But FMS can make you extra sensitive to any kind of pain and make ordinary sensations painful.

Lupus

Almost anyone who has lupus experiences achy joints, a low-grade fever, and extreme fatigue—all symptoms you see in fibromyalgia. But lupus is an autoimmune disorder that occurs when the body's immune system attacks its own cells and tissues. For reasons that no one knows, the body cannot tell the difference between foreign substances and its own healthy cells and tissues.

Experts estimate there are 500,000 to 1.5 million Americans who have been diagnosed with lupus. No one knows what causes the immune system to go awry. Only about 10 percent of people who have lupus have a parent or sibling with the illness, and only about 5 percent of children born to parents with lupus eventually develop it. That's why the environment is believed to play a role in the onset of lupus. Possible environmental triggers include infections, stress, antibiotics, ultraviolet light, and hormones.

Lupus can strike at any age, and occurs in both men and women, though women are ten to fifteen times more likely to get it.

Types of Lupus

Lupus is difficult to diagnose. To make matters even more complicated, there are actually three kinds of lupus:

Systemic Lupus Erythematosus (SLE)

Systemic lupus erythematosus (SLE) can affect almost any organ or system in the body. This chronic inflammatory condition alternates between flares and periods of remission. SLE is by far the most common form of lupus. It is also the most serious form, and in extreme cases it can be fatal.

Discoid Lupus

Discoid lupus is a less serious form of lupus that is limited to the skin and causes a rash on the face, neck, and scalp. About 10 percent of cases will become systemic lupus.

Drug-Induced Lupus

People who take certain medications may wind up with drug-induced lupus. Drugs that can provoke a bout of lupus include hydralazine, which is used for hypertension, and procainamide, which is used to treat irregular heart rhythms. This condition occurs only in about 4 percent of people who take these drugs and goes away when the drug is discontinued.

Symptoms and Diagnosis

More than 90 percent of people with SLE experience joint and/or muscle pain, brought on by inflammation or arthritis. Many also suffer fatigue, rashes, anemia, and sensitivity to light. Some develop a butterfly-shaped rash across the cheeks and nose. In addition, symptoms may include Raynaud's phenomenon, hair loss, and involvement of the kidneys.

Diagnosing lupus involves the presence of four of the following eleven symptoms:

- Rash over the cheeks
- Red raised patches on the skin
- Sensitivity to sunlight, resulting in rash or increase in rash
- Ulcers in the mouth or nose
- Arthritis pain in two or more joints
- Inflammation of the lining of the heart or lungs
- Excess protein or other abnormalities in the urine
- Seizures or psychosis
- Low red or white blood cell count
- Positive antinuclear antibodies (ANA) in the blood
- Positive auto-antibody tests

Many of these symptoms may not occur at the same time. Some may come and go or simply change. As a result, getting a diagnosis of lupus can sometimes take months, even years.

Fact

Women who have endometriosis are at greater risk for autoimmune disorders, such as lupus and rheumatoid arthritis, as well as chronic fatigue and immune deficiency syndrome and fibromyalgia. Endometriosis is a condition characterized by the overgrowth of tissue in the abdominal cavity. It affects approximately 8 to 10 percent of women in their childbearing years.

Treating Lupus

The goal of treatment is to prevent flares, treat them appropriately when they occur, and minimize damage to body organs. Treatment often involves a cocktail of medications that may include nonsteroidal anti-inflammatory drugs, antimalarials, corticosteroids, and immune suppressants. Just as the disease will change over time, so too will the treatments.

How Lupus Differs from FMS

Although lupus and fibromyalgia are two distinct illnesses, it's not unusual for people to have both conditions. Among people who have lupus, approximately 10 to 40 percent also eventually develop fibromyalgia.

At times, it may be difficult to distinguish lupus from fibromyalgia, especially if you have FMS and are only suffering from pain and fatigue. But while lupus and FMS have those symptoms in common, there are definite differences between the two conditions, most notably in the blood and urine.

Lyme Disease

In the mid 1970s, a cluster of children in Lyme, Connecticut, experienced what they thought was an outbreak of juvenile arthritis. But the cause was eventually traced to a bacterium called *Borrelia burgdorferi*.

Lyme disease is transmitted by deer ticks that become infected by feeding on small rodents. When an infected tick bites a human or animal, it can pass along the bacterium, which then travels into the bloodstream and causes a number of symptoms, some of which can be quite severe. Within days or weeks, the infected person may develop a bull's eye rash around the site of the bite and a flu-like illness.

Anyone who lives, works, or spends time outdoors in areas where deer live is at risk for Lyme disease. Your best way to prevent Lyme is to avoid these areas such as overgrown fields or dense woods. Deer ticks generally lurk in places within three feet off the ground, including leaves, plant stems, and grass, but they can also be found in well-kept lawns and gardens.

Symptoms and Diagnosis

It may be days or weeks before the first symptoms of Lyme infection emerge. In about 80 to 90 percent of cases, you will see an expanding rash that usually radiates from the bite. On some people, the rash may resemble a bull's eye. In dark-skinned people, the rash may look more like a bruise. About the same time, you may experience flu-like symptoms, such as joint pain, fever, chills, and fatigue. Although bothersome, these symptoms may not be severe. They may even disappear, only to recur later.

As the disease progresses, the symptoms may become more severe. You may experience a stiff neck, facial paralysis, severe fatigue, numbness, and tingling. Weeks or months later, you may develop severe headaches, painful arthritis, swelling of the joints, cardiac abnormalities, and neurological problems characterized by memory loss, disorientation, and confusion.

Determining whether you have Lyme disease is usually a two-step process. Many patients are first given an enzyme-linked immunoassay (ELISA) test first. The ELISA can detect elevated blood levels of antibodies produced in response to the *Borrelia burgdorferi* bacterium. The ELISA is most effective if it's done at least four weeks after a tick bite.

But people who do not have Lyme disease still sometimes test positive, which is why all positive ELISA results are confirmed by the Western blot test. The second test looks for more specific Lyme antibodies in the blood. The combination of the ELISA and Western blot is currently considered the best diagnostic tool for detecting Lyme disease.

Alert

Not all ticks are infected with Lyme disease. And most ticks don't start transmitting the disease until an average of thirty-six to forty-eight hours after they've attached themselves. Your best bet is to find ticks before they can infect you. Scan your body after an outing in tick-infested areas. If you do see a tick, remove it by its head with tweezers, firmly and steadily without twisting.

Treatment

Caught early, the disease can be almost always effectively treated with antibiotics, which may be given for as long as four weeks. In cases that involve arthritis, a second course may be prescribed. Antibiotics may be given orally or by injection.

How Lyme Differs from FMS

There's no doubt that Lyme disease can resemble fibromyalgia. Both conditions cause muscle aches, numbness, and fatigue, and both can resemble arthritis. In the later stages, Lyme can cause the cognitive problems that resemble fibro fog.

A diagnosis of Lyme, however, does not necessarily rule out the possibility of fibromyalgia. In some people, having Lyme disease can be the traumatic event that triggers the onset of fibromyalgia. But getting an accurate diagnosis is important. Long-term treatment with antibiotics for people who have fibromyalgia and not Lyme disease will not relieve FMS. In fact, such treatment can cause troubling gastrointestinal side effects and make you resistant to subsequent antibiotics.

Hypothyroidism

The butterfly-shaped thyroid gland is located just below your Adam's apple, at the front of your neck. This vital gland is part of the endocrine system and churns out hormones that dictate how your body uses energy—which is your metabolism—namely thyroxine (T4) and triiodothyronine (T3).

People whose bodies produce inadequate amounts of thyroid hormone develop hypothyroidism. Women are more prone to hypothyroidism than men, especially after the age of forty. Experts estimate that 20 million people in the United States have hypothyroidism.

The most common cause of hypothyroidism is an autoimmune condition called Hashimoto's thyroiditis, in which antibodies attack the thyroid and damage it, reducing its ability to produce hormones. Other causes include radiation treatments, medications, and thyroid surgery. Hypothyroidism may also be caused by a malfunction of the pituitary gland, which releases a hormone called thyroid-stimulating hormone (TSH). TSH regulates the production of thyroid hormones.

Symptoms and Diagnosis

Hypothyroidism typically causes fatigue, weakness, and joint or muscle pain, especially in the shoulders and hips. Women who have it are susceptible to depression and sensitive to the cold. They may also develop puffiness in the skin. Other symptoms include dry skin, brittle nails, hair loss, constipation, and irregular menstrual periods. Some women experience an increase in their cholesterol levels and gain weight.

Diagnosing hypothyroidism is based on a doctor's thorough examination as well as blood tests that measure levels of T4 and serum TSH in the blood. If your thyroid isn't making enough hormones, your pituitary will release more TSH in order to compensate for the shortfall.

Treatment

The goal in treating hypothyroidism is to restore the deficient hormone to its normal levels. To do that, patients are generally given additional thyroid hormone. You will receive treatment the rest of your life, but it's important to monitor your hormone levels. The dosage of your medications can vary, depending on changes in your hormones.

 Alert

Women who have a hypothyroid have another reason to quit smoking. Studies show that women who smoke had higher levels of LDL, the bad cholesterol, as well as higher total cholesterol levels, both risks for heart disease. The smokers also had more muscle problems. Cigarette smoking apparently impairs the secretion and action of thyroid hormone.

How Hypothyroidism Differs from FMS

It's easy to see why hypothyroidism is sometimes confused with FMS. The widespread aches and fatigue are symptoms of both conditions. But simple blood tests that measure hormone levels can determine whether an underactive thyroid is the culprit. Interestingly, many people who thought they had fibromyalgia have seen their symptoms completely disappear when they were later diagnosed with and treated for hypothyroidism.

Rheumatoid Arthritis (RA)

Waking up to stiff and achy joints is the bane of all arthritis sufferers. But for about 2.1 million people in the United States, the pain is the result of rheumatoid arthritis (RA), an autoimmune disease in which the immune system mistakenly attacks the healthy lining of the joints.

Fact

Rheumatoid arthritis has afflicted some of history's most successful people, including the French impressionist painter August Renoir, who tied a paintbrush to his arthritic hand in order to continue painting. Other famous folks with RA include Christiaan Barnard, the first surgeon to perform a heart transplant, and actresses Lucille Ball and Kathleen Turner.

No one knows what causes the immune system to attack the joints. Although scientists have confirmed that RA is linked to a cluster of genes, not everyone who carries these genes will get the condition. At the same time, not everyone who gets RA carries these genes. That's why experts believe that it's probably a combination of genetic susceptibility and environmental triggers that causes RA. Possible triggers may include infections, stress, cigarette smoking, and occupational hazards. And since 70 percent of all people with RA are women, experts suspect hormones may play a role.

Rheumatoid arthritis can be extremely painful, and in severe cases, it can be disabling and life altering. The condition is chronic, but the pain can ebb and flow, depending on life circumstances, medications, and stress. It can also go into remission.

Symptoms and Diagnosis

People who have RA typically have morning stiffness in and around the joints. They may experience arthritis in three or more joint areas, and the arthritis may afflict the hands. In addition, the arthritis may occur symmetrically, meaning that if a joint on the right side hurts, the same joint on the left side will hurt, too. Some people will also feel lumps under their skin, called rheumatoid nodules.

Diagnosing RA is based on a doctor's examination, blood tests, and imaging studies. Blood tests may show the presence of certain substances in the blood, including rheumatoid factor, anti-cyclic citrulline-containing peptides (CCP) antibodies, and antinuclear antibodies (ANA). X-rays, CAT scans, and MRIs may reveal erosions or decalcifications in or around the affected joints. Usually, it's a combination of these measures and the patient's own self-reported symptoms that lead to a diagnosis of RA.

Treatment

Treating RA is an imprecise science that may require experimentation. Patients often wind up taking several drugs, including nonsteroidal anti-inflammatory drugs, disease-modifying anti-rheumatic drugs, and biologic response modifiers. Some of the medications are very powerful and can have profound effects on your immune system.

How RA Differs from FMS

RA and fibromyalgia might feel similar, and the symptoms may be described in the same way. But the two conditions are really rather different. RA is primarily a disease of the joints, while FMS pain can occur anywhere. RA actually causes damage to the body, while FMS does not physically injure you. Blood tests and imaging scans can help pinpoint whether you are suffering from RA.

Other Conditions

Many other conditions can also mimic fibromyalgia. In fact, any condition characterized by pain and fatigue could potentially be mistaken for fibromyalgia or vice versa. Among them are those described in the following sections.

Osteoarthritis

More than 20 million people in the United States have this degenerative condition, making it the most common cause of physical disability. In osteoarthritis, the cartilage that cushions bone gets eroded, leaving bone to rub against bone. The resulting pain can restrict movement and also cause fatigue, swelling, and stiffness.

Multiple Sclerosis (MS)

Multiple sclerosis (MS) is thought to be an autoimmune disorder in which the body attacks its own nervous system. This causes widely varying, inexplicable neurological problems that can come and go without apparent cause. Symptoms vary and can change from time to time, but may include fatigue, weakness, tremors, loss of balance, bladder and bowel problems, and depression.

Polymyalgia Rheumatica (PMR)

Polymyalgia rheumatica (PMR) is an arthritic condition that causes your muscles to feel achy and stiff. The discomfort is brought on by inflammation triggered by an autoimmune response. The inflammation usually occurs in the hips and shoulders, but it can be elsewhere, too. The condition is most common in adults over age seventy, especially women.

Mononucleosis

Mono, or the kissing disease, as it's commonly called, is an infection caused primarily by the Epstein-Barr virus. It typically produces flu-like symptoms such as fatigue, fever, body aches, and sore throat. The symptoms usually last about four weeks and go away on their own, but in some cases the virus remains in your body for life.

CHAPTER 4

Finding the Right Doctors

Long before you got sick, you probably went to a doctor once or twice a year for a checkup. Now that you have a chronic illness, you'll need to become more serious about the doctors you choose. Not only do you need skilled health professionals, but you also need ones you like, who believe in you and your condition, communicate well, and address your needs. This chapter will help you identify the health-care people you might need (and want) on your team.

Team Captain: You

Having fibromyalgia typically means you'll need more medical attention than you did in the past. It may also create emotional and psychological issues that you've never experienced, and it can involve treatment options that often seem confusing. And if you're already wracked with pain and fatigue, you might find it hard to muster the energy to even locate the right medical help.

But the first thing to remember in selecting your doctors is that you're the boss. Doctors, family, and friends may provide referrals, but it's ultimately up to you whether you'll use that person's services. Being the boss also means you have to be assertive about your needs. So if you've always felt uncomfortable talking to your primary care doctor or disliked the office location, now is the time to do something and find someone new.

The key to spearheading any team is knowing what you want. Do you want someone whose office hours match your work hours? Does the office location make a difference? Do you prefer young doctors fresh out of medical school or doctors who've been in practice for several years? The answers to these questions can help you zero in on the doctors who will make up your team.

Question

Help! How can I learn to take charge?
If the idea of spearheading anything gives you the willies, relax. Being in charge simply means looking out for your care. If necessary, practice assertiveness skills with a friend. Try speaking "I" messages, as in, "I didn't like how that medicine made me feel."

Who Are the Key Players?

Not everyone who has fibromyalgia has the same type of doctors or health-care specialists. The physicians you see will depend on the symptoms you are experiencing and whether you can get satisfactory answers. A person who has irritable bowel syndrome, for instance, will need the expertise of a gastroenterologist, while a psychiatrist might be involved in treating depression.

When it comes to finding good doctors, it's critical to find those who acknowledge the reality of fibromyalgia. Many people, including those in the medical community, still don't believe that fibro exists. It doesn't seem to matter to them that fibromyalgia has been recognized as a bona fide medical problem by the World Health Organization, American Medical Association, and the American College of Rheumatology. These people still think that fibromyalgia is "all in your head." But when you're in pain, the last thing you need is a health-care professional who disregards your complaints and treats them as hogwash.

It's also important to find doctors who are on top of the most current studies on fibromyalgia. Research into fibro is constantly evolving, and modern medical knowledge moves at a rapid clip. A doctor who stays on top of what's new is more likely to provide you with the best and most up-to-date care.

Finally, you want health-care professionals who are compassionate and understanding. Granted, not every good doctor is blessed with good bedside manners, and good technical expertise can usually compensate for a lack of warmth. But a caring physician can make it more appealing for you to go to the doctor. The following sections describe some of the key players you'll need.

Fact

Prepare for your first appointment by reading, "Choosing a Doctor," a pamphlet written by the Agency for Healthcare Research and Quality. The pamphlet is available on the Internet at *www.ahcpr.gov/consumer/qntascii/qntdr.htm*. It offers information on everything from how to talk to your doctor to how to check his credentials.

The Primary Care Doctor

Whether it's your long-time family doctor, an obstetrician-gynecologist, or an internist, the lead doctor is your primary care doctor. This person is the one you summon first when you don't feel well or a new symptom emerges. The primary care doctor is the first person to evaluate your problems and determine whether they need further investigation. They often screen new symptoms to determine whether they are due to FMS or another condition. If it is another condition, they will determine which treatments should be provided. This doctor is also the "quarterback" of your team and will decide when you need to see a specialist, help steer you to the best, and coordinate the activities of your various treatment providers.

The Lead Doctor (Your "Fibrodoc")

The lead doctor should be familiar with fibromyalgia or, at the least, have a desire to learn more about it. He could be your primary care doctor or a specialist, such as a rheumatologist, endocrinologist, physiatrist, or pain management doctor. Your fibrodoc might even be a chiropractor. The next sections describe health-care professionals who are most likely to treat people with fibromyalgia.

Rheumatologist

Many people with fibromyalgia wind up seeking out a rheumatologist. Rheumatologists specialize in the diagnosis and treatment of autoimmune disorders such as lupus, rheumatoid arthritis, and scleroderma. But they also treat people who have arthritis and musculoskeletal conditions, osteoporosis, and sports-related injuries.

After four years of medical school, and three years of training in internal medicine, rheumatologists spend another two to three years in rheumatology training. Most choose to become board certified, which requires passing a rigorous exam conducted by the American Board of Internal Medicine.

While in training, rheumatologists learn the skills it takes to become the medical detectives that their field demands. Unlike some doctors who focus on certain organs—such as neurologists, who treat brain disorders—rheumatologists treat conditions that involve numerous organs and body systems. They must also learn to read X-rays of joints and to understand the ways numerous medications work in the body.

But a skilled rheumatologist doesn't end his training with medical school or board certification. A good rheumatologist will stay on top of all the research and developments in medicine.

Family Practice Physician

Family physicians treat the whole person and the person's family. They do not restrict their practice to a certain age group, the way geriatricians do. And they don't confine their practice to one gender, the way obstetrician-gynecologists do. They're also not restricted to focusing on one particular organ or body system, the way cardiologists concentrate on the heart and the circulatory system.

Although the field is general in its scope, family practice still requires specialty training. After graduating from medical school, family physicians complete a three-year residency program and participate in inpatient and outpatient learning. They also receive training in pediatrics, obstetrics and gynecology, internal medicine, community medicine, surgery, psychiatry, and neurology. In addition, they are taught about several other aspects of medicine, including geriatrics, ophthalmology, radiology, orthopedics, and urology.

 Fact

At the beginning of the twentieth century, 80 percent of all U.S. doctors were in general practice. By 1969, when the field of family practice was created, only 50 percent were generalists. Today, there are nearly 70,000 practicing family physicians in the United States. They make up 12 percent of all patient care physicians in the United States and are part of the 41 percent involved in primary care.

Internist

Doctors who treat adults are called doctors of internal medicine or internists, which is not the same as a medical intern in training to become a physician. Those who specialize in the nonsurgical treatment of diseases of the internal organs are known as internists.

These doctors devote their medical school training to the prevention, diagnosis, and treatment of diseases that affect adults. They are generally well rounded in their knowledge and are equipped to treat common problems involving the eyes, skin, ears, nervous system, and reproductive health. They are also expert at knowing when to defer to specialists when problems become complex. But they often remain involved in coordinating a patient's care. Internists who choose to pursue a subspecialty, such as cardiology, oncology, or infectious disease, go on to receive additional education and training.

Osteopathic Physician

Doctors of osteopathy (DOs) are just like medical doctors (MDs). They must complete four years of medical education and follow up with an internship and residency program. They often serve as primary care doctors and are able to prescribe medications and perform X-rays. They're licensed by states according to individual state regulations.

What makes DOs different from MDs is that their training emphasizes viewing the body as an integrated whole, with the whole being greater than the sum of its parts. Although MDs are taught this same lesson, there is less emphasis on the integrated approach to the body in traditional medical schools. Rather than just treat the symptoms affecting one body part or system, a DO will treat the whole person. The belief is that once the body is functioning properly, it can heal itself.

Osteopathic medicine also puts greater emphasis on prevention and health maintenance. Their treatment methods reflect that philosophy and may incorporate hands-on manipulation of bones and muscles, a procedure known as osteopathic manipulative treatment. These manipulations can be used to diagnose injury and illness, improve blood flow, and promote healing.

Fact

Osteopathy is not alternative medicine, though it was once considered quite radical. It was founded in 1874 by a physician named Andrew Taylor Still. Although initially regarded with skepticism, his ideas eventually took hold. In 1892, he started the American School of Osteopathy in Kirksville, Missouri. Today there are twenty colleges of osteopathic medicine—including the A.T. Still University in Kirksville—with nearly 10,000 students.

Obstetrician-Gynecologist (OB-GYN)

Some women with fibromyalgia turn to a trusted OB-GYN for their initial health problems. OB-GYNs are trained in the medical and surgical care of women, and they specialize in issues regarding reproductive health, including pregnancy, childbirth, and disorders of the reproductive system. They provide screenings of sexually transmitted diseases, preventive tests for breast and cervical cancers, and assistance with family planning.

Although OB-GYNs are not trained specifically to deal with FMS, they do treat women, who make up the bulk of people with fibromyalgia. Because of this, some OB-GYNs take the time and effort to learn a great deal about fibromyalgia. They may also be enlisted if someone with FMS develops vulvodynia or any other problem involving reproductive health.

Pediatrician

Children who are diagnosed with fibromyalgia may be under the care of a pediatrician. Pediatricians who cannot treat FMS may be able to refer your child to a pediatric rheumatologist or another specialist.

Other Specialists You Might Need

The health-care professionals discussed so far are the most likely ones to serve as your primary fibromyalgia doctors. But for people who have fibromyalgia, the symptoms can affect a variety of body systems, and their needs may require the attention of other specialized physicians.

Endocrinologist

Endocrinologists specialize in treating the body's endocrine system, which regulates hormones. Hormones are essential substances produced by different glands, and they are involved in everything from reproduction to metabolism. An endocrinologist may be consulted to treat problems such as thyroid disease, diabetes, endometriosis, and infertility.

Neurologist

Anyone who endures inexplicable pain is a candidate for the neurologist's office. Neurologists specialize in diagnosing, treating, and managing disorders of the brain and nervous system, which includes pain and pain management. Some neurologists may focus on treating patients with Alzheimer's, multiple sclerosis, or Parkinson's.

Physiatrist

Any injury that might require rehabilitation could fall under the scrutiny of a physiatrist. Physiatrists specialize in physical medicine and work to restore function to injured muscles and joints. Some physiatrists may even specialize in fibromyalgia. Physiatrists also treat people who have suffered strokes, neurological disorders, and multiple sclerosis.

Psychiatrist

Sometimes, the emotional problems caused by fibromyalgia can become serious. That's when you might need a psychiatrist. Psychiatrists are medical doctors who specialize in the treatment of mental illness and emotional problems. Unlike psychologists, psychiatrists can perform laboratory tests and medical tests that offer a complete picture of your well-being. They can also prescribe medications or offer psychotherapy.

Pain Management Specialist

It's not unusual for the pain of fibromyalgia to become so severe that your other doctors become uncomfortable managing it. In some cases, specialized procedures such as an epidural injection are required to reduce it. Or there may be so many medications involved that it requires the knowledge of someone who specializes in their use. Pain management doctors have extensive training in all the types of procedures and medications that can help relieve pain.

Physical Therapist (PT)

People who are suffering from extreme pain or need help with physical recovery may turn to a physical therapist (PT) for assistance. PTs work with patients to develop a physical treatment plan that addresses their pain in order to improve a patient's independence and self-sufficiency.

A PT may use numerous techniques to reduce your pain, including exercise, hydrotherapy, electrical stimulation, heat, and cold. After getting an assessment and doing a physical exam, the PT will work with you to devise a program of rest and exercise that improves your function. The exercises are designed to strengthen your muscles, improve your range of motion, and enhance cardiovascular conditioning. They can also provide casting and splinting and educate patients on proper body mechanics.

 Fact

In a 2005 Canadian study published in the *Clinical Journal of Pain*, researchers found that fibro patients who had multiple rehabilitation strategies felt better than those treated just by their family physician. The multidisciplinary group was treated by a rheumatologist and physical therapist and had supervised exercise therapy, as well as massage therapy. They also heard lectures on pain and stress management and diet.

Occupational Therapist (OT)

In the midst of fibro pain and fatigue, even the simplest tasks can seem daunting. That's where the occupational therapist (OT) can help. OTs are the most practical of medical professionals. They typically get involved when a patient has trouble getting through the routines of daily life.

OTs work with patients to help them learn how to move through their routine in ways that cause less pain. The OT also helps you find ways to conserve energy so that you never overexert yourself. In addition, an OT can help you find the splints and equipment you need to protect your joints, reduce your pain, and improve your function.

Pharmacist

Before you got sick, you probably had few encounters with a pharmacist. But if you have fibromyalgia, you may require more medications than you needed in the past. Having a good relationship with a pharmacist can become important to your health. So choose a pharmacist you like and trust, and use that person for all your prescriptions.

⌐, Essential

Any medication can have side effects, especially if taken with another food or substance. Calcium-rich foods, for instance, lessen the effectiveness of some antibiotics. Gingko biloba, an herbal remedy, can interfere with blood clotting if you're on aspirin. Decongestants can cause blood pressure to spike in people who take antihypertensive medications. Read all labels carefully, and discuss anything you take with your doctor or pharmacist.

Pharmacists can provide a wealth of information, some of it lifesaving. The pharmacist can alert you to potentially dangerous drug interactions and possible side effects from any medications you're prescribed. He can tell you whether an over-the-counter remedy or herbal supplement will interact with a prescription medication you're taking. He can also advise you on whether drugs require food before they're ingested.

There is also a pharmacy specialist called a pharmacologist. These are pharmacy-trained professionals who specialize in helping patients who must take numerous or unusual medications. The pharmacologist helps them deal with dosing patterns and avoid drug interactions, as well as other challenges. Since some patients with severe fibro might wind up on a number of medications, a pharmacologist may be called on to coordinate their use.

Psychologist

Living with a chronic illness that is potentially disabling can cause a constellation of emotional and psychological symptoms such as anger, depression, fear, and anxiety. Patients may also experience difficulties in their personal relationships, work situations, and families.

A psychologist can help you work through these myriad issues through counseling and therapy. After a thorough discussion and evaluation of your problems, a psychologist can help you devise the coping skills you need to overcome these difficulties. Since stress aggravates FMS, a psychologist can also teach you mind-body techniques that enhance relaxation and bolster your pain management.

Social Worker

Social workers may get involved in a person's life on several levels. They may provide counseling and help locate services in the community that aid in a patient's recovery. They can also identify resources that address a patient's need for financial help, home care, transportation, and support groups.

For the unfortunate people who are unable to work as a result of FMS, a social worker can help them navigate the social services maze in order to secure assistance.

Finding the Best Doctor

Locating a good doctor is important for people with fibromyalgia. Dealing with the medical profession can be stressful, confusing, and time-consuming, which can exacerbate the pain you're already experiencing. A good doctor can make all the difference in how you fare, so choose carefully and deliberately.

Studies have shown that the best form of care for fibromyalgia patients is a multidisciplinary program incorporating several different forms of care in one clinic. At this time, there are very few multidisciplinary fibromyalgia clinics in the United States. But if there is one in your area, you should definitely check it out.

Where to Find a Doctor

In an era of managed health care, insurance companies often dictate the doctors we see. After all, few of us can afford to pay for health care that isn't covered by an insurance plan. The good news is that most plans today have numerous doctors, even in subspecialties. But in reality, a name on a list tells you very little about the doctor.

Essential

Looking for a physician in your area? Check out the American Medical Association's Physician Select at *http://dbapps.ama-assn.org* and enter your state and zip code. The site also tells you where the doctor went for medical school, where he did his residency, and whether he's certified in his specialty. You may also find a physician through the National Fibromyalgia Association at *www.fmaware.org*.

To locate a primary care doctor, ask friends, neighbors, colleagues, and family for recommendations. Talk to people who have fibromyalgia and find out who they see. An excellent source is a support group. Members have experience with health-care providers in your area and can guide you to those who are "fibro-friendly."

When you need a specialist, you may get a name from your primary doctor, which is sometimes good enough. But if you don't like the doctor, check around with friends and family again, or go back to your primary doctor for another recommendation.

Interview the Doctor

Whether you're selecting a primary care doctor or another health-care specialist, it's important to do some research before deciding to go to a physician on a regular basis. Even if the doctor comes to you as a recommendation from your best friend, you may find him unsuitable in ways that don't bother your friend. Ideally, you should take time to meet the doctor and do your own assessment or interview.

Some good questions to ask yourself and the doctor include the following:

- Does the physician specialize in the treatment of FMS?
- Does he already have patients with fibromyalgia?
- What kinds of alliances does the physician have with other health-care professionals or hospitals?
- Are there other people in his practice who can assist in your care?
- What kind of health insurance does the doctor accept?
- What kind of communication skills does the physician have? Do you feel comfortable in his presence?
- Would it upset the doctor if you sought a second opinion?
- What does the doctor think of alternative therapies?
- Does he listen to what you say and answer your questions in words that you understand? Does he call back when you need assistance or information?
- How convenient is the office to your home or workplace?

Don't underestimate the importance of the office support staff. Schedulers, nurses, and assistants who are courteous and respectful can make a big difference in how well you do with your doctor. A bad encounter or stressful office visits can cause undue stress, which will only worsen your fibromyalgia symptoms.

What to Expect from a Good Doctor

When you choose a doctor to treat you for fibromyalgia, you should look for someone who first and foremost believes that your symptoms are real and that FMS is a bona fide medical condition. The doctor should also have confidence in finding relief for your symptoms. She should be well versed in the subject of fibromyalgia and should stay on top of research by reading medical journals.

She should also be an effective communicator who can speak to you in comprehensible terms without resorting to medical terminology to explain what she means. At the same time, she needs to be a good listener, even when you're questioning her or telling her you'd like a second opinion. She should always invite you to ask questions and offer ideas.

Alert

Having fibromyalgia or any chronic disease makes you vulnerable to quackery. Be wary of any doctor who promises you quick relief, a special remedy, or even a cure. Treating fibromyalgia takes time and a great deal of trial and error. So if something sounds too good to be true, it probably is.

Finally, a good doctor should be open, honest, and forthcoming with information. He should be willing to provide you with any report or information you want, even if he's afraid the news is bad.

Steer clear of any doctor who is remotely skeptical of fibromyalgia or your symptoms. A doctor who doesn't believe you will only make your symptoms worse. Also, avoid those who are always in a hurry or reluctant to give you the time you need. And of course, do not go to doctors who don't make you comfortable. Your health and well-being depend on your ability to be frank and forthcoming. Any physician who makes you uncomfortable will not encourage open communication.

The First Visit

Once you've located the right doctor, you will need to make time for a thorough exam and evaluation. Make sure to set aside enough time for this appointment so you won't feel rushed. This first visit is critical to helping your doctor make a diagnosis and determine your need for specialists. Most important, it will set the tone for the future of your relationship. Here are a few of the things you can expect at this first visit:

- A frank and thorough discussion of your symptoms, when they began and where you hurt

- A detailed medical history of you and your family
- Descriptions of any changes in your health, such as changes in appetite, sleep patterns, weight loss or gain, and cognitive function
- Questions regarding recent events in your life that may have caused undue stress
- Discussions about your lifestyle, including diet and exercise habits, and your consumption of drugs and alcohol

A thorough physical examination will also be done to determine whether your symptoms are the result of something besides FMS. During the exam, a doctor familiar with fibromyalgia is almost certain to do palpations to pinpoint the location of your tender points, since this is how fibromyalgia is diagnosed. Palpation of other tissues can also help distinguish fibromyalgia from myofascial pain. In addition, your doctor may order blood work and urine tests to determine whether you have another condition.

Essential

Sometimes your gut instinct is as good an indicator as any other measure of whether someone is trustworthy or not. So trust your inner voice if a doctor gives you bad vibes, even if she is giving you all the rights answers, accepts your health insurance, and offers office hours that match your schedule.

Leading Your Team

Now that you've assembled a team, you have to continue serving as its leader. That means staying on top of what's going on. A big part of that job is keeping good medical records. Doctors see hundreds of patients a year, and it can be difficult for them to keep track of which patient takes which medication or when they last saw a certain patient. When it comes time to see you, they'll rely on what you tell them to help them figure out what to do next.

Your Medications

Always keep an updated list of all medications you take, including the dosages and when you take them, along with the names and numbers of your physicians and any drug allergies you have. It's a good idea to keep a copy of this list on your computer so you can update it easily if you need to.

You should also keep a separate list of every medicine you have ever tried for FMS, including the dosage used and why you stopped using it. This can be very helpful to your doctor, since it can guide him away from trying certain families of medications that haven't been helpful or that caused side effects in the past.

Any Doctor Visit

Record all your doctor visits in one place, even dental checkups. Write down the purpose of your visit, any symptoms you were experiencing, and any medications or therapies you were prescribed. Also record your height, weight, and blood pressure.

Consultation Reports from Specialists

Any time you see a specialist, ask for a report of the visit. These typed narrative reports provide comprehensive descriptions of your symptoms, of what happened during the exam, and of any lab findings. The specialist may also offer an analysis of the problem and a plan of action.

Lab Tests

Whenever your doctor orders blood work or an X-ray, make sure to ask to get copies, too. Although you can't detect fibromyalgia in these tests, they do give indications about the status of your health. Over time, they can give you clues about how your health is changing. If necessary, give the receptionist a self-addressed stamped envelope to ensure you get the information.

Preventive Screenings

When you have a chronic condition, it's important to keep track of all medical information, even preventive screenings that show you are healthy. Down the road, that information can establish a pattern. For instance, even if your bone density tests are still in the normal range, they can, over time, reveal a decrease in density that may show you to be at risk for osteoporosis. So get in the habit of tracking the results of your preventive screenings—such as mammograms, Pap smears, and bone density tests—by asking the receptionist to send you a copy of the results.

Discharge Summaries for Hospitalizations

If you're hospitalized, the attending physician will write up a summary of your visit, the procedures you underwent, the diagnosis, and your health status. If you have an outpatient procedure, ask for an operative report, which details your visit.

Communicate!

As the team captain, you also have to keep lines of communication open on all levels, even between doctors. For some people, that might mean being more assertive and outspoken than you have been in the past. If that makes you uneasy, try writing down your questions and concerns in advance, which can also save time.

Just as you want your doctor to speak clearly to you, so too should you be open and clear with her. Ask questions whenever you're uncertain. Listen closely to what your doctor tells you, even taking notes if necessary. If you don't like a treatment she suggests, say so and ask for alternatives. Good communication will form the foundation of a successful relationship with your medical team.

CHAPTER 5

Diagnosing Fibromyalgia

Getting a diagnosis for fibromyalgia is somewhat like assembling a complex puzzle. Putting together the pieces takes time, patience, and the keen eye of a skilled and observant physician. If you're in the throes of pinning down a diagnosis, this chapter can help you figure out how the experts identify this mysterious condition and whether you do have fibromyalgia.

The Official Word

Unlike other conditions, fibromyalgia cannot be measured or seen on X-rays, blood tests, or biopsies. That's why getting a diagnosis for fibromyalgia has always been so difficult. Although further delving has proven that fibro sufferers do have chemical differences—such as increased spinal fluid levels of the neural hormone substance P (a compound that increases pain sensitivity)—those tests are costly and currently restricted only to research.

For years, fibromyalgia was diagnosed purely on the subjective report of the patient. That is, the doctor made a diagnosis based on what the patient told him. In fact, the condition didn't even have a distinct name until the 1980s. Although descriptions had been documented in medical texts for centuries, the condition was known by other names such as fibrositis, chronic rheumatism, chronic muscle pain syndrome, and psychogenic rheumatism.

In 1980, a group of physicians got together and set out to create an official way to define fibromyalgia. They broke up into two groups and evaluated patients who had complained of widespread pain and who had also been told by their physicians that they did indeed have fibromyalgia.

Not surprisingly, symptoms varied widely. The most common finding between the two groups was widespread pain, with fatigue and sleep problems close behind. One clear finding was that the patients were much more tender to even light touch than normal people. As a result, the researchers chose eighteen specific spots to test for this type of tenderness. If the spot hurt when the doctor pressed on it—just hard enough with his thumb to make the nail turn white—it was considered a positive tender point. Among patients who had fibromyalgia, nearly 89 percent had widespread pain and sensitivity in at least eleven of the eighteen tender points. Although the effort was initially meant to make it easier to classify fibromyalgia for the purposes of research, these findings eventually became the diagnostic criteria set by the American College of Rheumatology.

Essential

Adults aren't the only ones to develop fibromyalgia. Children may have juvenile primary fibromyalgia syndrome. The symptoms resemble those in adults, with stiffness and fatigue being the primary complaints. If your child has fibromyalgia, explain it to her in simple terms—"The Princess and the Pea" is a good story to use. Most importantly, find a doctor who knows how to treat it. For help, contact the American Juvenile Arthritis Foundation, a branch of the Arthritis Foundation, at www.arthritis.org.

The American College of Rheumatology Criteria

You're wracked with pain, but is the pain bad enough to qualify for a diagnosis of fibromyalgia? According to the American College of Rheumatology (ACR), an organization that focuses on diseases involving the muscles, tendons, or joints, the pain must be widespread—on the left and right sides of the body, above and below the waist. The pain should also have been present for at least three months.

In addition to widespread pain, a diagnosis of fibromyalgia requires that you be tender in at least eleven of eighteen tender point sites. These sites are all around the body in specific locations. To make matters even more precise, the pain must be felt during digital palpation, which means pain is caused when an examiner applies 4 kg/cm^2 of force—the equivalent of eight pounds—to the tender point, just enough pressure for the health-care provider's fingernail to turn white. The tender points occur on both sides of the body and above and below the waist. For an illustration of the tender point locations on your body, check out the ACR description of fibromyalgia at *www.rheumatology.org*.

Other Telltale Signs

While the ACR criteria are the formal measure for determining whether you have fibromyalgia, they are by no means the only indicators. For instance, you might have only eight tender points but be achy all over and suffering from poor sleep. You may also have memory problems, morning stiffness, and irritable bowel syndrome. Some FMS sufferers experience chronic headaches, joint pains, and swelling.

In the quest to pin down a diagnosis, a good doctor will ask you about these symptoms. How are you sleeping? Are you stiff when you wake up? Where else do you hurt? If the doctor doesn't ask, take the initiative and tell him. The more information you provide, the better equipped your doctor is to make a diagnosis.

Just because you may not qualify for a diagnosis of FMS doesn't mean you shouldn't be treated. People can have nine tender points but be miserable with pain, fatigue, and sleep disruption. Whether or not you qualify for the label of fibromyalgia is not the most important issue. Instead, the goal of treatment should be to make life livable again. The same treatments used for fibromyalgia can probably help you, even if you don't fit the strict diagnostic criteria.

A Tough Diagnosis

Now that you know the guidelines for diagnosing fibromyalgia, you may be wondering why it's so hard to figure out whether someone has this perplexing condition. After all, no one would complain about widespread pain if they didn't have it, and tender points are so specific that it seems it should be easy to determine if someone has FMS. But in reality, there are several reasons why fibromyalgia is hard to diagnose.

Changing Symptoms

The primary signs and symptoms of fibromyalgia are fairly specific, but the symptoms may crop up at varying times. It's quite possible for you to feel pain at numerous tender points at one doctor's visit and then experience relief at a follow-up appointment a month later. That's because the disease itself is characterized by periods of flareups and remission. In other words, the telltale signs and symptoms don't have to occur at the same time for you to have fibromyalgia.

Deceiving Appearances

People who have fibromyalgia look healthy. In fact, you may appear to be completely well, even when you're in the throes of mind-numbing pain. Fibromyalgia causes no outward deformities or changes in the joints and muscles, and people with fibro do not look sickly. About the only outward sign of poor health might be dark circles under your eyes, caused by the lack of sleep.

Fact

Even the nineteenth-century inventor and industrialist Alfred Bernhard Nobel had a hard time convincing people he was ill. But a 1996 review of his letters to his mistress showed that Nobel—the inventor of dynamite and creator of the prestigious prize for intellectual achievement—probably had fibromyalgia. He complained of sleep disorders, unrelenting pain, and paralyzing fatigue. His family thought he was a hypochondriac, and his letters suggest he could not find relief despite visits to elegant European spas.

While no one complains about looking good, some patients might consider their healthy appearance a source of frustration. Even close friends and family members may find it difficult to believe that you're sick. It's not uncommon to hear well-meaning friends say, "But you look great." In fact, it's not uncommon for family, friends, bosses, and even some physicians to accuse fibromyalgia patients of faking their pain.

Sadly enough, there are those who do in fact fake fibromyalgia. Some people looking for drugs, sympathy, disability, and workman's compensation have unscrupulously pretended to have fibromyalgia. Unfortunately, since there is no test that can prove they *don't* have fibro, many of these people get what they wanted. Fears over these fraudulent cases have made every fibro patient suspect in the eyes of employers and even many doctors.

Everyone's Different

When it comes to fibromyalgia, no two patients are alike. Some may have only lower back pain and occasional bouts of insomnia. Others may be in such extreme pain that they are wheelchair-bound. Some people experience tender points in places other than the eighteen identified by the ACR. The fact that patients differ so widely in their symptoms only causes more confusion and makes it hard for doctors to determine whether someone has fibro.

Too Many Imitators

As you've already read in Chapter 3, fibro has many imitators. These fibro imitators can make it hard for doctors to figure out which condition you have and even whether you have more than one. Usually, physicians do rigorous testing to rule out other conditions before making a diagnosis of fibromyalgia. But even if you test positive for something else, it doesn't mean you don't have FMS. Fibromyalgia is not a diagnosis of exclusion.

With so many imitators, patients can spend as many as five years trying to track down a diagnosis. Others may spend years mistakenly believing they have something else. Consider the case of Nan.

For twenty years, Nan's doctors told her that she had rheumatoid arthritis. The diagnosis frightened her. She thought for sure that by the time she turned forty, her body would be wracked by deformities and that she'd be living in a wheelchair. But when doctors examined her after a car accident, Nan was told she had fibromyalgia. Nan found the news to be a great relief and now looks back on the car accident as a blessing. She has since been able to relieve her pain with yoga, tai chi, and meditation.

Misplaced Blame

It's easy to attribute the symptoms of fibromyalgia to lifestyle factors. Chronic fatigue may simply be the product of too many late nights at the office. Your aches and pain might be the result of advancing age. Poor sleep and fatigue are likely byproducts of demanding responsibilities. None of these assumptions is unrealistic, and for millions of people, these symptoms really are a matter of lifestyle. But if your initial symptoms are mild, and you attribute them to lifestyle factors, you may wind up delaying a diagnosis and proper treatment.

Medical Skepticism

Even with the support of prestigious medical groups such as the World Health Organization, the American Medical Association, and the ACR, too many doctors remain unconvinced that fibromyalgia is a real medical problem. They may believe the condition is the product of stressed-out patients who can't cope with the rigors of life. Or they think fibromyalgia is a psychosomatic disorder, the result of a person prone to depression, anxiety, and psychological distress.

Working with medical professionals who do not believe fibromyalgia exists is a major impediment to getting accurately diagnosed and treated. Of course, not all doctors will tell you that they don't believe in fibro. That's why it's important for you to be able to spot a nonbeliever and to then find a doctor who considers fibromyalgia a bona fide medical problem.

New Criteria

It's been a mere fifteen years since the diagnostic criteria for fibromyalgia were established by the ACR. That means some doctors still in practice today were never trained to spot the signs and symptoms of fibromyalgia. They also may not really understand the condition.

Getting to a Diagnosis

Now, you may be wondering how anyone is ever diagnosed with fibromyalgia when there are so many obstacles to a quick and accurate diagnosis. That's why it's so important to choose a doctor you like and trust, someone you believe will do her best to work toward a diagnosis. That takes time and patience, and it helps to know that your physician is in your corner.

Truth is, there's often nothing quick about getting diagnosed with fibromyalgia. Patients often undergo a lot of testing and waiting. In the meantime, you may be dealing with remarkable pain and fatigue while awaiting an answer. Hopefully, though, your doctor will start you on treatment while waiting to confirm your diagnosis.

Even though there are no markers in the blood or images on an X-ray to reveal you have fibromyalgia, your doctor will still need to order tests and examine the findings to rule out other conditions. Here is what you can expect in the process.

Getting an Answer

The diagnostic process usually begins the minute you show up at your doctor's office. It typically starts with a conversation about your current lifestyle, what you do for a living, whether you have children, and why you've come to see the doctor. Your doctor will also inquire about medications and supplements you are taking, whether you exercise regularly, and whether you drink alcohol or smoke cigarettes.

From there, your doctor should begin to ask you about your current symptoms. What exactly are you feeling? When did the pain begin? Was there something that happened to cause your discomfort? What have you tried to relieve your symptoms, if anything?

Be sure to tell your doctor everything, even if it might seem embarrassing at first. For instance, you may not want to discuss your vaginal pain during sex or your frequent trips to the bathroom throughout the day. But such symptoms may be revealing. Vaginal pain may be vulvodynia, and frequent urination may signal irritable bladder, both conditions associated with fibromyalgia.

Alert

Unfortunately, doctors are often quick to brand fibromyalgia patients as difficult patients, especially if the doctor is skeptical. You can help lessen that image by being calm, organized, and specific about your symptoms. Also be realistic. Don't expect your doctor to diagnose you immediately. If you sense he isn't taking you seriously, then by all means go elsewhere. But do present yourself credibly and calmly.

In addition to your current problems, your doctor will ask about your medical history as well as that of your family. It's a good idea to ask family members beforehand whether they've experienced similar symptoms or health problems. Again, speak frankly and openly about your family's medical past. A history of depression, while embarrassing to your mother, is nothing your doctor hasn't heard before. Such details can help your doctor determine the source of your problems since many medical conditions have a genetic component.

Your doctor will also want to know what kinds of events have been happening in your life recently. Have you recently been in a car accident? Are you happily married? Have you gone through any major changes in your life, such as moving or switching to a new job? Events that might lead to fibromyalgia include the following:

- Grief that has gone on for six months or longer
- Injuries related to a car accident
- Recent illness or infection
- Repetitive movements and misuse of muscles

Other possible culprits include depression—which could be the result of your problems, not a cause—allergies, immobility, overworking, and nutritional deficiencies. Information about recent events in your life may lead to other questions that can reveal stressors that might have triggered your symptoms.

Testing, Testing

Most experts agree: A good fibromyalgia doctor today now knows well enough to do a digital palpation test, which is an important diagnostic tool specifically for fibromyalgia. Be sure to tell your doctor if the palpation hurts when she applies pressure. Just because a site is uncomfortable does not mean it is truly painful, and it is the presence of pain that defines fibromyalgia.

In order to rule out other medical problems, you will still need to undergo other kinds of testing. For starters, your doctor will probably order a complete blood count. Although fibromyalgia does not reveal itself in blood markers, blood does give you a snapshot of your overall health. Blood tests can also reveal an iron deficiency (anemia) and antibodies that show whether you may have an autoimmune disease. In addition, blood provides information on how well your kidneys and liver are functioning.

Other kinds of tests your doctor orders will depend on your symptoms. These might include, but are not limited to those described in the following sections.

Infectious Disease Tests

If your symptoms resemble those of Lyme disease or another infectious disease, your doctor may subject you to tests for these conditions. For Lyme disease, for instance, you may need the Western blot and ELISA tests.

Thyroid Tests

If your physician thinks hypothyroidism is behind your symptoms, she may ask that the lab check your thyroid hormone levels during your blood test.

Imaging Tests

X-rays, CAT scans, or MRIs are sometimes ordered if your doctor suspects compression of your spinal cord by a disk or rheumatoid arthritis. These imaging studies can detect damage around the affected joints.

Sleep Testing

Some people who complain of extreme fatigue may be suffering from sleep apnea. Sleep apnea is serious. If it's severe, it can even be fatal, so diagnosis and treatment of this condition is important.

Question

Why not test for substance P?
Several studies have determined that people with fibromyalgia average three times more substance P in their spinal fluid than healthy people. But it's hardly a conclusive diagnostic tool. Some fibro patients have normal levels, and elevated levels are also present in people who have osteoarthritis and chronic back pain. Getting tested for substance P also isn't easy and requires a spinal tap.

Testing for sleep apnea typically involves an overnight stay at a sleep clinic, where a polysomnography is done to record the number and duration of apnea episodes in a given night. (A polysomnography is a diagnostic test that involves sleeping in a study center where several measurements are taken simultaneously while you sleep, including respiration, eye movement, and brain wave activity.)

Even if it turns out you don't have sleep apnea, a sleep test can help identify whether you are getting the deep restorative sleep that many fibro patients lack. It can help your doctor assess your sleep quality and then prescribe medicines to correct the problem.

How You Can Help

The best medical treatment requires a strong partnership between you, the patient, and the doctor, the expert. When it comes to medical conditions such as fibromyalgia, which rely heavily on what patients reveal, a doctor is most effective at diagnosing your problem if you are open and honest about your symptoms, lifestyle, and medical history. Being shy, coy, stoic, or dishonest is not a good approach toward securing an accurate diagnosis. As the patient, there are also other steps you can take to help make the diagnosis process a little easier, such as the following:

- Offer as much information as you possibly can, with as many details as you can remember.
- Go in prepared with a list of questions and concerns.
- If possible, write down the medications you take ahead of time. Include the dosages and how long you've been taking them.
- Write down any medications or over-the-counter remedies you've tried in the past, along with the reason you're no longer taking them.
- Bring a notebook so you can take notes on what the doctor tells you.
- Be on time. Doctors are busy. If you're late, that cuts into the time your physician can spend working with you.

Also, learn as much as you can about fibromyalgia. Knowledge is power when it comes to your health. Knowing what the doctor should look for can help move the process along, especially if your doctor has had little experience with fibromyalgia.

Dealing with Nonbelievers

Doubters may infuriate and frustrate you, but no one is more problematic than the physician who doesn't believe. After all, you're turning to the doctor for an answer and relief from your symptoms. While it isn't always easy to escape doubters among friends, family, and colleagues, you can make the choice to dump your doctor. There is absolutely no reason or obligation for you to continue to see a doctor who isn't addressing your problems or trying to uncover the reasons for your suffering. Do your research. Check with friends and acquaintances and find a new doctor. The trouble will be well worth it in the end.

If you get really frustrated by people who don't believe your condition is real, there are tests that can be done. Qualified psychologists can do a battery of tests that can tell whether you're suffering psychological consequences (such as stress) from a real medical illness, or getting medical symptoms from psychological problems. Showing the results to nonbelievers can go a long way toward convincing them that your suffering is real.

When You're Diagnosed

The good news is that recent research and articles on fibromyalgia have finally started to validate the reality of this condition. When you finally hear that you have fibromyalgia, you may actually be relieved. After months and possibly years of probing, you have an explanation for the chronic pain, poor sleep, and the myriad other symptoms you may be experiencing. Now that you have a name for your symptoms, you can begin the process of trying to reverse the pain and fatigue, taking control of your health, and going on with your life.

CHAPTER 6

All about Pain

Long before you learned you had fibromyalgia, you'd already known pain. You felt it when you got a splinter in your finger or twisted your ankle playing sports. You felt pain when you jammed your toe into the dresser or sliced your finger on a piece of paper. But according to people who have fibromyalgia, the intensity of the pain that comes with FMS is unlike anything you might have felt before. Because pain is at the core of fibromyalgia, it helps to understand the concept of pain itself.

What Exactly Is Pain?

As uncomfortable as it is, pain is your body's built-in alarm system. When your body is injured or afflicted with disease, nerves transmit signals to the brain, which we in turn translate as pain. Pain is undoubtedly unpleasant, but it does warn you that something is awry. The signal may be telling you to pull your hand away from the hot stove or to avoid walking until a leg fracture heals. It's nature's way of preserving your body from further damage.

The extent of your pain depends primarily on what occurred that started the sensation. Certainly the prick of a pin is a much milder form of pain than a hammer on your thumb. It also depends on how much pain you can tolerate, which is highly subjective. Other factors that influence your pain threshold include your mood, your temperament, and whether you had a good night's sleep.

℧ Question

Is pain the fifth vital sign?
Most doctor visits involve measuring your blood pressure, pulse, respiration, and temperature—what medical experts have for years called the "vital signs." These indicators help doctors gauge a patient's health and aid in the diagnosis and treatment of disease. Increasingly, doctors are recognizing that pain is also a way to assess health and well-being, another vital sign.

The Nervous System

In order to understand why we feel pain, it's important to know a little about the body's nervous system, an elaborate network of nerves whose control center is the all-important brain. The nervous system is the body's most complex system and regulates hundreds of activities—all at the same time.

At the center of the nervous system is the brain, which is the root of your consciousness, the center of your intellect, and the basis of your creativity. The brain also regulates your autonomic processes, all those things your body does that don't require a moment of conscious thought, such as breathing, blinking, and heart rate.

The nervous system is made up of several distinct parts, each with several unique roles. Think of it as a collection of electrical wires and impulses, all activated and regulated by the brain.

The Central Nervous System (CNS)

The central nervous system (CNS) is made up of the brain and the spinal cord. The brain is the hub of all information processing and bodily functions, while the spinal cord links the peripheral nervous system to the brain. The brain controls reflexes and is the initial pain processing center. The brain, which weighs all of about three pounds, is nestled securely in your skull, where it houses about 100 billion neurons, or nerve cells, that are constantly transmitting information among cells. It is the place where all impulses originate and where all impulses travel. Absolutely everything we do, from casting a nasty glance or laughing at a joke to reading a book or learning a musical instrument, requires our brain.

 ## Fact

Over time, many luminaries have sounded off on pain. Leonardo da Vinci and his contemporaries came up with the idea that the brain was the main organ responsible for sensation and that the spinal cord was the part that transmitted pain. The poet Emily Dickinson said pain had "no future but itself." The twentieth-century French missionary Albert Schweitzer described pain as a "more terrible lord of mankind than even death itself."

The Peripheral Nervous System (PNS)

The peripheral nervous system (PNS) is an elaborate network of nerve fibers that branch out from the brain and spinal cord to the far reaches of your body, such as your fingertips. This network has the vital task of constantly receiving information from inside and outside the body, then relaying that information to the brain to find out what to do. The PNS is made up of two parts.

The Sensory Somatic Nervous System

Swallowing, chewing, a wiggle of your toes. All these tasks are performed by the sensory somatic nervous system. This system kicks into gear, either voluntarily or involuntarily, when your senses are stimulated by external stimuli such as food, texture, and sound, or by conscious desires, such as when you want to move.

The Autonomic Nervous System

Anything involuntary that we do is regulated by the autonomic nervous system. Blinking, breathing, and digestion are all processes regulated by this system. It also alerts us to danger, tells our intestines to digest our food, and responds to our emotions.

How Nerves Cause Pain

The nerves, which are located throughout your body, are the sites where you first receive impulses and also the site where you start to process and transmit them. In fact, nerves are the starting point of your pain.

L. Essential

It isn't easy to describe something as subjective as pain. One way to do it is to use a numeric scale of 1 to 10. A verbal scale describes the pain as mild, moderate, or severe. Children might use the Wong-Baker scale, which uses faces to describe degrees of pain. You can also help your doctor's understanding with words like "radiating," "excruciating," or "dull," or by describing where your body hurts, how the pain affects your activity, and whether anything makes it worse or better.

At the ends of the nerve fibers are nociceptors, receptors that detect actual or potential tissue damage. Millions of these nociceptors lurk in your skin, bones, joints, muscles, and in the membrane that surround your internal organs. Nociceptors are most prevalent in regions that are prone to injury, such as your fingertips and your toes, or in critical sites such as your eyes.

When these nociceptors sense that something has hurt your body, they immediately transmit a signal to your brain in the form of an electrical impulse. The impulse travels along the nerve to your spinal cord, where it enters a region called the dorsal horn. There, the signal sets off the release of chemicals called neurotransmitters, which then activate other nerve cells that process the information and send it up to your brain.

Making Sense of the Information

Once in the brain, the information arrives in the thalamus, which serves as the brain's information relay system. All sensory information passes through the thalamus. The information is processed and prioritized and is then sent to multiple parts of the brain:

- The somatosensory cortex, or physical sensation region
- The limbic system, or emotional feeling region
- The frontal cortex, or thinking region
- Deep brain structures that control processes including blood pressure, pulse, and hormone release

These multiple pain messages explain why we respond to pain on several levels. When your finger touches a thorn on a rose bush, your brain might react by saying "Ouch, it hurts," "I never did like roses," and "Move that finger!" all at once.

Fact

A 2004 survey of 1,039 employees at a *Fortune* 100 company found that 29 percent of respondents had pain problems that affect work performance. The workers with pain scored 45 percent lower on ratings of their physical health and 23 percent lower on measures of mental health. Those in pain were five times more likely to report health-related limitations on their ability to do their job.

At the end of this split-second transmission, the brain has the task of interpreting the message and deciding what to do with this new information. This decision depends on your age, the circumstances, and your life experience. A child who receives pain signals from a thorn, for instance, may cry and run for her mother. A woman at a party may stifle the urge to cry out and simply inspect and stroke her finger. A gardener may pause and seek relief by placing ice on the injury. How a person chooses to respond depends in large part on the memories stored in the brain, which tell her how effective her previous responses were, as well as what the person has been taught about how to respond to pain.

Normal Pain Versus Fibro Pain

Pain is a normal part of the human experience, but what about pain that seems to serve no purpose, like the widespread musculoskeletal aches that afflict people with fibromyalgia? To better understand the difference between normal pain and the pain in fibromyalgia, we need to distinguish acute pain from chronic pain.

Acute Pain

The bothersome toothache that signals a cavity. Throat pain that alerts you to a strep infection. The agony of a broken leg in a skiing accident. These are examples of acute pain, which usually results from a recent injury or disease. Acute pain grabs your attention and demands you take action. But once it's properly treated, the pain disappears, and you recover.

Chronic Pain

If acute pain—or its cause—isn't treated quickly, the nerves "learn" to be in pain. Changes occur within the nerves and their surrounding structures that cause the pain to persist. If these changes become severe enough, the pain will persist even after the cause has disappeared. Acute pain then turns into chronic pain.

People with fibromyalgia suffer chronic pain, often severe enough that it pervades their very existence. In fibro, the pain is not always preceded by a traumatic event—though sometimes it is—and the injured tissue may appear perfectly fine. So while chronic pain may be telling you that something is wrong, it's often difficult to pinpoint the problem.

Chronic pain can persist for months, even years. Acute pain that recurs over and over again is also called chronic pain. Typically, people who have chronic pain have fewer treatment options because the source of the hurt is often in the nervous system itself. That's why people who have conditions such as fibromyalgia often speak of managing their pain.

What Causes Fibro Pain?

Truth is, no one really knows exactly what brings on the aches and pains of fibromyalgia. What we do know about fibro pain is that it involves a complex interplay of highly sensitive nerve fibers known as C-fibers and the rest of the central nervous system.

Essential

It's hard to imagine that beauty products might cause pain. But a Swedish researcher found a possible link between cosmetics and pain. The study, which involved forty-eight women with FMS, found that using less makeup and following a special skin-care regimen resulted in diminished pain, better sleep, and improved physical function. While hardly conclusive, the study suggests that cosmetic use might impact fibromyalgia symptoms.

Everyone has small C-fibers in the skin. These slow-moving nerve fibers are highly sensitive to chemical, mechanical, and thermal energy. Your tongue for instance, may react to both the chemical and thermal energy of hot chili peppers. Overstretching a muscle, on the other hand, is a mechanical stimulus for pain. When these stimuli are strong enough, they activate the C-fibers. The C-fibers send their information to pain-processing nerve cells in the spinal cord, which then pass their information up to the brain. If stimulation of the pain fibers is too intense or goes on for too long, a condition known as central sensitization occurs. Central sensitization is a condition in which neurons in the central nervous system become overexcited and normal sensations become abnormally painful. Sensations that come from C-fibers in the muscles are more likely to trigger central sensitization than input from the skin.

Central sensitization results in wind-up phenomenon, in which your response to pain is significantly increased. In essence, the computer that processes pain in your spinal cord becomes hyperactive. You become overly sensitive to heat. A tap on the arm feels like a punch. The soft texture of a cotton blanket makes you ache.

When the wind-up phenomenon occurs, other nerve fibers that don't normally carry pain start to get involved in the transmission of pain signals in order to handle the overload of stimulation. Now more nerves are charged up.

In this excited state, the body becomes hypersensitive to pain. For some people with fibromyalgia, even a warm bath is enough to cause bodily distress. When mildly painful events become very painful, you are said to have hyperalgesia. When a person feels pain due to a stimulus that would normally not cause pain, it is called allodynia.

Pain Without Stimulus

In some cases, people experience pain without any input or stimulus. This seemingly bizarre phenomenon occurs when people feel pain in the absence of any external factor, such as injury. It's caused by spontaneous discharging of the nerves that normally carry or process pain, often due to some type of irritation or injury. The classic example is phantom limb pain. A patient whose left leg has been amputated, for instance, might still complain that his left ankle hurts. Phantom limb pain may seem impossible, but it lends further proof to the fact that people can feel pain even if they haven't suffered any obvious trauma, just as fibro patients do.

Body Chemicals Involved in Fibro Pain

In people who have fibromyalgia, certain body chemicals are altered, which can affect the degree of their pain. In addition to central sensitization and wind-up phenomenon, changes in the levels of certain neurochemicals in your body can exaggerate your sensitivity. Some of the neurochemicals involved in fibromyalgia include substance P, serotonin, endorphins, and growth hormone.

Substance P

People who have FMS have higher-than-normal levels of substance P, a chemical that makes pain nerves much more sensitive. High levels of substance P make a person quicker to feel pain than someone with lower levels. Studies show that people with fibromyalgia have, on average, about three times the normal level of substance P.

Research has also shown that simply applying pressure to bring on pain does not appear to increase substance P levels. This finding suggests that elevated levels of substance P aren't brought on by something external but rather that something internal is raising the levels.

Serotonin

Serotonin is a neurotransmitter found in unusually low levels in people with fibromyalgia. Neurotransmitters are chemical messengers that transmit messages through nerve cells. Serotonin has numerous roles in the body. It regulates mood and alleviates depression, promotes sound sleep, and relieves pain. It also regulates the immune system and promotes smooth muscle function.

Endorphins

Most times when you get hurt, emotionally or physically, your body doesn't sit by idly and absorb the assault. It launches its own defense. One way that it does that is by releasing natural opiates called endorphins. These feel-good substances are also responsible for the high that some people experience from exercise, sex, addictive drugs, and certain foods, such as chocolate.

Endorphins block the transmission of pain within the nervous system by binding to the same receptor sites that pain signals use. But in people who have chronic pain like fibromyalgia, endorphins offer little respite. After a while, enzymes called endorphinase devour the endorphins, rendering them ineffective.

Growth Hormone

Low levels of serotonin and other hormones, a lack of deep sleep, and overproduction of a compound called somatostatin cause many fibro patients to have abnormally low levels of growth hormone, a substance essential to normal muscle metabolism and repair. A reduction in growth hormone occurs in about a third of fibromyalgia patients.

 Alert

Researchers at the University of Michigan have found that women are better able to tolerate pain when estrogen levels are high by releasing endorphins that soften the signals. Unfortunately, a dip in estrogen, which occurs just before your period, reduces the system's effectiveness, which may explain why women say their FMS symptoms are worse during their periods.

As much as 80 percent of growth hormone is secreted when we are in the deepest stages of sleep. If we are deprived of deep sleep—which is what happens in fibromyalgia patients—the muscles go unrepaired. Even tiny microtraumas go unrestored and are subject to further damage. Low levels of growth hormone usually also result in low levels of insulin-like growth factor (Ig-4), another hormone. While some studies have shown that giving growth hormone to correct the deficiency can reduce fibro symptoms, the treatment costs almost $80,000 a year, and most insurance plans won't pay for it.

The Gate Control Theory

One day, you shriek at the slightest paper cut. The next day, you gouge your finger on a knife and continue chatting with your friend. Has your pain threshold changed overnight?

In the 1960s, two psychologists devised a theory of pain that helped to explain why pain sometimes appears and disappears, seemingly without rhyme or reason. The gate control theory says that as pain signals travel to the brain, they pass through nerve gates that can be opened or closed. When the gates are open—as they are when you're tired, stressed, or depressed—pain messages pass through more readily. When they are closed—by way of relaxation techniques, drugs, or heat, for instance—the messages are blocked. If you have fibromyalgia, it's important to understand what opens up your pain gate. Likewise, it's just as critical to identify strategies and factors that can close your pain gates. Even though the amount of pain may be the same, you may be able to alter your perception of it and reduce its impact. Your interpretation may be affected by several factors, including the following:

- **Memories of previous pain**—Did that paper cut hurt you in the past?
- **Upbringing**—If your parents stressed the importance of grinning and bearing pain, you may be trained to withstand more duress.
- **Beliefs and value system**—You despise wimpy people who cry out at the slightest pain, so you refuse to do the same.
- Attitude—Those who hate the dentist are more apt to feel the pain of the drill.
- **Expectations**—You don't anticipate that a fall will hurt, so it doesn't.
- **Age**—Falling off a bike may have seemed like a minor event when you were a kid but now causes excruciating pain for you as an adult.
- **Sex**—Because they are trained to "be tough," men may be groomed to feel less pain.
- **Social and cultural influences**—Unspoken cultural influences may affect your tolerance for pain.

Changing some of these factors can make a big difference in how you perceive pain. But it isn't always easy to change long-held beliefs and expectations. Doing so requires a strong desire for change, as well as practice and patience.

Impact of Lifestyle

Exactly what causes the body's response to pain to intensify in fibro-myalgia patients remains a mystery. It's also still unclear why various hormones and substances become elevated or deficient. Until scientists develop a better understanding of these factors, there is little we can do to affect these bodily functions so that fibro pain is reduced or eliminated.

Fact

When it comes to sympathy for chronic pain sufferers, family members are the best source of comfort, while bosses are the worst. A 2003 survey by Peter D. Hart Associates found that 75 percent of pain sufferers got support and help from significant others and family members. But 16 percent said their bosses were downright indifferent and tended to ignore them when the topic of pain came up.

But there are things in your life that you can control that will make a difference in your pain. The kinds of food you eat, the exercise you get, the emotions you feel, and the amount of stress in your life are all factors that can affect the degree of your pain. Happy people who eat well and exercise regularly (without overdoing it) are less likely to experience intense pain than those who eat poorly, are emotionally distraught, and get no exercise.

What often happens with pain is that you wind up trapped in a vicious cycle, one that you must break if you are to regain some semblance of control. Here's how it might go:

- Something goes wrong inside your body that exaggerates your pain response.
- Chronic pain ensues.
- Sleep becomes difficult, if not impossible.
- You become too tired to do anything, and your muscles lose their conditioning.

- As a result, you become depressed, which only makes your pain worse.

And on and on it goes.

Interrupting this cycle of pain is important for people with fibromyalgia. Maybe you can't silence your demanding boss or find a less exhausting route to the office each day. But you can eat a better diet, get more exercise, and change the way you perceive these stressful events so you're less upset. Doing so can make an enormous difference to your health and well-being.

Good Nutrition

While no single diet has been found to improve or worsen pain, many people notice that certain foods can affect the degree of their pain. Some people, for instance, get a headache from eating too much chocolate. Others find it soothing. But almost everyone with fibromyalgia should avoid the sweetener aspartame (most commonly marketed under the brand name NutraSweet). Aspartame contains a compound called aspartate. In the body, aspartate is easily converted to a neurotransmitter called NMDA, which stimulates pain fibers.

 Alert

Some people with fibromyalgia may notice a craving for carbohydrates. The urge to load up on carbs is often the result of exhaustion, depression, and low levels of serotonin. Unfortunately, for many fibro patients, refined carbohydrates may actually worsen their symptoms, though they might not notice until the next day.

If you've identified specific foods that seem to exacerbate your pain, then obviously you should steer clear of them. What you should eat, however, is less clear in terms of pain relief. In general it's always best to eat a healthy, well-balanced diet, one that helps you maintain your weight and steer clear of disease. That means eating a diet that is rich in fruits and vegetables and whole grains, and low on fat, cholesterol, sodium, and sugar.

Exercise Matters

The thought of doing any sort of exercise when you're in pain might seem daunting, even impossible. But being inactive perpetuates the cycle of pain and causes muscles to become increasingly deconditioned.

Getting regular exercise, albeit painful at first, can actually lessen your pain. Regular activity also releases feel-good endorphins into your bloodstream, promotes restful sleep, and boosts serotonin levels. In addition, it reduces depression, enhances your immune system, and, over time, can improve your self-esteem and your feelings of control over your condition.

The key is not to overdo it and to avoid injury. Keep your expectations reasonable and realistic. If you can do only five or ten minutes at first, then do that without attempting to do more. The goal is to exercise regularly and to establish it as a habit.

Hurtful Emotions

Negative emotions can affect the amount of pain you feel on any given day. In fact, experts now believe that pain is not just a tactile sensation but an event that is strongly connected to the emotional centers of our brains. It creates an emotional response to something going wrong inside the body, much the same way emotions can be reactions to events occurring outside the body.

Research is showing that our emotions have a great deal to do with the pain we feel. Dwelling on our pain with anguish and frustration typically makes it worse, while distraction can provide relief. Studies have found that pleasant odors that improve our mood can diminish pain, while noxious ones that worsen our mood can increase our pain.

The connection between emotions and pain suggests that efforts to control our feelings can relieve our pain. The challenge, however, is that persistent pain and poor sleep naturally cause feelings of despair, anger, and sadness, even in the most resilient people. But doing our best to counter these feelings is well worth the effort. For more information on managing your emotions, see Chapters 15 and 16.

The Stress Connection

In small doses and certain situations, stress is a good thing. A case of performance anxiety, for instance, can make you work harder to polish a big speech. The sound of someone breaking into your house in the middle of the night can heighten your senses and prepare you to flee. The stress of being on time for an appointment might make you leave your house a little earlier.

But chronic stress is unproductive and can cause all sorts of health problems, including a worsening of your pain. Chronic stress can cause you to gain weight, abandon healthy habits, and lose sleep. In people who have fibromyalgia, stress can make your pain even worse.

Essential

Next time you're feeling sad, angry, or frustrated, take some time to pamper yourself. A little self-indulgence can help ease negative emotions, and it doesn't have to be a costly. A cup of tea by the fireplace, a walk with your significant other, or a chat with an old friend are all simple things that make you feel a little better. The key is to do something that takes your mind off the negative emotions you're experiencing.

As anyone who has fibromyalgia knows, having fibromyalgia alone can be a source of stress. The frustration of trying to get a diagnosis and attain relief can rattle the nerves of even the calmest person. And the unpredictable nature of the condition can worsen the stress. Not knowing how you will feel days or weeks from now can make it hard to plan your life.

Just as a lack of exercise can put you on a vicious cycle toward more pain, so too can the effects of stress. The cycle goes something like this:

- You have fibromyalgia.
- It causes stress, which is compounded by the hassles of daily life.
- The result is more stress, which increases your pain and fatigue.

And on and on it goes, until you're besieged by pain, fatigue, and stress.

That's why taking control of stress should be a part of any pain management plan. Whether the stress comes from your condition, your family, or any other area of your life, it's important to keep it in check. Sure, you may not be able to put a stop to your boss's controlling behavior or your children's endless spats. But changing the way you react can make a world of difference in alleviating your stress and minimizing your pain.

Poor Sleep

In short, the worse you sleep, the worse your pain. That's because your body rebuilds, restores, and rejuvenates its tired muscles while you sleep. For fibromyalgia patients, however, quality sleep is often difficult to attain.

The best thing you can do for yourself is to try and practice good sleep hygiene. Go to bed at the same time every night. Get up at the same time every morning. Learn to relax and unwind before bed, and do not keep the television or computer in your bedroom.

Chapter 7

The Fatigue Factor

Everyone wrestles with feelings of fatigue at one time or another. Before a big exam. The morning after too little sleep or a late night out on the town. But for people with fibromyalgia, fatigue can be overwhelming, all-consuming, and frustratingly inexplicable. For some people, fatigue can be even a bigger problem than the pain. In people with fibromyalgia, fatigue seems to be an entity all its own.

Fibro Fatigue

The fatigue experienced by fibromyalgia sufferers is unlike ordinary fatigue, the kind you get from pulling an all-nighter or from dealing with a stressful spell at work. It is much more than just feeling tired from not getting enough sleep or from overexerting yourself. The kind of fatigue that people with FMS have is debilitating and comes out of malfunctions in your body's energy-producing processes. In some people, the fatigue can be life altering, forcing job changes and the end of beloved hobbies and activities. Unfortunately, even a good night's sleep does little to erase the agony. Here's how Connie describes her fatigue.

> "Fibro fatigue feels much like the flu without the sore throat," she says. "But the overall feeling is like the exhaustion you feel with the flu. Even little things can tire you out, like cleaning your shower, or going to the grocery store." To help relieve her fatigue, Connie carefully schedules all her daily tasks. She also tries to really listen to her body, and to rest whenever her body tells her it needs a break.

In short, fatigue is a state of mental and physical exhaustion that can impair your ability to perform daily activities. For people with fibromyalgia, fatigue may be worsened by the effort they put forth simply to do all the things that normally come so easily to them. There are actually three different types of fatigue affecting people with fibromyalgia:

- Mental fatigue, more commonly known as fibro fog, is characterized by low motivation and difficulties with focus, concentration, and judgment.
- Physical fatigue is the inability of the muscles to perform high-energy or repetitive activity. Physical fatigue, in particular, is a major reason why some people with severe fibro have to go on disability.
- Sleep-related fatigue is the exhaustion that comes from poor sleep.

Fatigue—especially physical fatigue—is a huge problem in fibromyalgia. Estimates show that as many as 75 percent of all patients experience fatigue. In fact, many people say fatigue is a bigger problem than pain. While we have medicines that can effectively treat pain and mental fatigue, we have nothing to treat physical fatigue. At their worst, people who have fibromyalgia-related fatigue can barely survive a trip to the supermarket. They cannot walk for extended periods or focus on tasks that require concentration. Even the slightest activity saps their energy. Barbara remembers a bad bout of fatigue while shopping in a department store.

Barbara was on her way upstairs, only to discover a long line at the elevator because the escalator wasn't working. So she joined the other shoppers in walking up the escalator, which had been shut down. But for Barbara, the trek up the escalator was exhausting. Every few steps, she stopped to rest and felt the overwhelming sensation that she was going to drop at any moment.

What Makes It Worse

Certain lifestyle factors and other medical conditions can make your fibro fatigue even more intolerable. One of the biggest culprits behind fatigue is the most obvious one: poor sleep. A bad night's sleep can make anyone tired the next day. But in people with FMS, sleeplessness can be a chronic problem. If you do sleep, the rest you get may be of such poor quality that you don't awaken refreshed.

⌐, Essential

> If you're suffering from severe fatigue, be on the lookout for depression. Constant fatigue can create feelings of frustration, sadness, and despair, making you vulnerable to depression. Major depression is a serious mental illness that warrants medical attention. It is characterized by persistent feelings of emptiness and lack of pleasure. If you suspect you have depression, consult your doctor immediately.

People who develop depression are also likely to have greater fatigue. Remember, having fibromyalgia already puts you at greater risk for depression. Once you're depressed, you may find you have even less energy.

In some people, the stress of having fibromyalgia can make the fatigue even worse. Juggling job, kids, and other responsibilities while battling fibromyalgia can put you on a collision course with stress. Over time, feeling constantly overwhelmed can exhaust even the heartiest souls. And the stress of having a challenging health problem will only make matters worse.

The foods you eat can affect your energy levels, too. When you eat a meal that is too high in carbohydrates, for instance, you may develop reactive hypoglycemia, a type of low blood sugar that occurs two to three hours after the high-carb meal. As a result, your body may secrete too much insulin, causing blood sugar to drop and signaling your body to release too much adrenaline. The result may be tremors, rapid heart rate, and sweating as well as mental confusion that can all compound your fatigue.

Alert

Many people use energy drinks for a quick pick-me-up. But most of these drinks are chock full of caffeine, sugar, or other substances that can leave you wired and awake later on, when you're ready for sleep. They can also be dehydrating. Mixing them with alcohol is potentially dangerous and can cause cardiovascular problems.

Over time, reactive hypoglycemia may result in insulin resistance. When that occurs, the body stops effectively using the insulin it produces. Since insulin is needed for sugar to get into your cells, this causes mild cell starvation, which also results in fatigue. The condition greatly raises your risk for diabetes.

Drugs can cause fatigue, too. Benzodiazepines and tricyclic antidepressants, for instance, can cause drowsiness and impaired memory. So can muscle relaxants, pain pills, and some antihypertensives. If you are taking medications that worsen your fatigue, talk to your doctor. She may be able to alter the dosage. You may also have to change the time of day you take the medication—from morning to night, for example—so that the fatigue is less disruptive.

CFIDS, a Co-conspirator

To make matters worse, some people with fibromyalgia also suffer from chronic fatigue and immune dysfunction syndrome, or CFIDS. It isn't easy to always distinguish one condition from the other. Some people with fibro may have symptoms of CFIDS, while others with CFIDS may experience the pains of fibromyalgia. The two conditions also share many other overlapping conditions, such as irritable bowel syndrome, depression, and cognitive dysfunction.

People who have CFIDS suffer from debilitating exhaustion and extremely poor stamina. They have problems with memory and concentration and often experience flu-like symptoms as well. One of the telling signs of CFIDS is how you fare after even the slightest exertion. Within twelve to forty-eight hours of any sort of physical or mental exertion, people with CFIDS typically experience a worsening of their symptoms and require an abnormally long period of time to recover.

Getting diagnosed with CFIDS isn't easy. To make matters worse, there are no blood tests, X-rays, or diagnostic markers that can help determine whether you have CFIDs. Instead, diagnosis depends on the patient's self-reported symptoms. For a list of criteria, see Chapter 3.

Essential

Be prepared for unexpected bouts of fatigue, which can strike at any time. Keep frozen meals and canned foods on hand. Make extra meals ahead of time, and store them in the freezer. When a bad bout of fatigue strikes, you'll at least have food available to feed yourself and your family.

Anyone can get CFIDS, but the condition is three times more common in women than it is in men. In women, it is more common than multiple sclerosis, lupus, HIV infection, and lung cancer. It can also occur, albeit rarely, in children and adolescents. In all, an estimated 800,000 people in the United States suffer from this mysterious condition.

Like fibromyalgia, no one knows exactly what causes CFIDS. But many people report the onset of symptoms shortly after a flu-like illness.

Could It Be a Virus?

In its earliest stages, CFIDS resembles the flu, with aches, fever, and chills accompanying the fatigue. These symptoms have prompted many scientists to question whether a virus is the infectious agent that triggers CFIDS.

In the 1980s, researchers thought CFIDS was brought on by the Epstein-Barr virus, the culprit behind the yuppie flu, only to later discount that idea after antibodies to the virus turned up in healthy people, too. Some scientists have since thought that CFIDS was the result of other viruses, such as the human herpesvirus6, a common virus that has been linked to multiple sclerosis and that lies dormant until reawakened. But that connection has not been firmly established in CFIDS.

Other microorganisms that have been suspected of causing CFIDS include mycoplasmas, a form of bacteria best known for causing walking pneumonia. Viruses linked to Coxsackie virus and polio have also come under scrutiny. But so far, researchers can find no solid evidence that CFIDS is caused by a specific virus.

Immune System Problems

Although no particular immune dysfunction has been singled out in people with CFIDS, research suggests that there may be abnormalities in the immune system that contribute to the symptoms. In most cases, the immune system of people with CFIDS appears to be weaker. A large percentage of people with CFIDS have also been found to carry autoantibodies, which suggests that CFIDS may be an autoimmune disorder.

Autonomic Nervous System (ANS)

The part of the central nervous system that controls your body's involuntary functions—such as heart rate, breathing, and digestion—may be faulty in people who have CFIDS. Studies have shown that people with CFIDS have trouble regulating blood pressure and are particularly susceptible to low blood pressure. Research has found that CFIDS sufferers are likely to faint when their bodies are tilted at a 60-degree angle.

Fact

Every time you move into a standing position, your body automatically undergoes a series of ANS reflexes that prevents blood from going down to your legs, which would cause you to pass out. Your diastolic blood pressure rises about 10 mmHg, and your heart rate goes up ten to fifteen beats. In people with orthostatic intolerance, these reflexes don't work properly, causing lightheadedness or fainting.

Another indicator of a link to the ANS is that a large number of people who have CFIDS also have orthostatic intolerance, an ANS-related condition in which changes in posture also cause dramatic changes in heart rate and blood pressure. The result is often dizziness upon standing and sometimes even fainting.

Too Many Cytokines

In people who have CFIDS, there appears to be an imbalance of cytokines, proteins produced by white blood cells that help regulate immune function. Many people with CFIDS have elevated levels of interleukin-1-alpha (IL-1 alpha), a type of cytokine that promotes inflammation. IL-1 is the same cytokine that causes the inflammation seen in rheumatoid arthritis. Other cytokines cause fatigue, which is why all you want to do when you're sick is lie in bed.

Thyroid Troubles

Many people who have fibromyalgia or CFIDS resemble patients with hypothyroidism. They're sluggish, slow, and prone to weight gain. They lack any energy and crave sleep. And yet tests show that their thyroids are functioning fine. Some doctors believe that people with

CFIDS or fibromyalgia have an abnormally low metabolism. Although the thyroid is churning out the right amount of hormones, the body is unable to recognize them. Since thyroid hormone increases metabolism, this malfunction results in less energy in the body cells.

Adenosine Triphosphate (ATP) Shortage

Some experts believe that people with CFIDS or fibromyalgia have a shortage of adenosine triphosphate (ATP). ATP, the body's primary source of fuel, is produced in the mitochondria of body cells. All carbohydrates, proteins, and fats from food are converted into ATP. When there is enough oxygen in supply, more ATP can be produced. But when oxygen is limited, the normal mechanism shuts off, and the body switches to a process called anaerobic glycolysis, which produces considerably less ATP and more undesirable byproducts. Think of the burning feeling you get when you're working a muscle really hard. That burn comes from the release of acids caused by anaerobic glycolysis. Experts believe that people with fibromyalgia have less oxygen in their muscles and reduced capacity for ATP production. The result? Fatigue.

Treating Fatigue

Unfortunately, treating fatigue is not easy. Antidepressants and hypnotics, for instance, may be prescribed to help promote sleep. Stimulants or anticonvulsants can sometimes relieve cognitive problems. Some herbal products, such as malic acid or ginseng, may help pick you up. If your fatigue is accompanied by gastrointestinal disorders, you may need an antispasmodic or antianxiety medication. Unfortunately, there are no medications just for physical fatigue.

Whatever medications you are prescribed, take them with caution. People with CFIDS often are unusually sensitive to medications and may need to start on lower-than-usual dosages. In some cases, your doctor may start you on doses below what is considered therapeutic and then gradually work up to a dosage that is of greater benefit. Also keep in mind that medications are not your only treatment option. In some cases, you might benefit from occupational therapy, which can teach you new ways of doing things. Physical therapy can help you with exercises that promote relaxation and reduce muscle tension. You should also consider meditation and other stress-reducing strategies, which can help relieve muscle tension as well.

Living with Fatigue

Unfortunately, for some people, fatigue is a constant companion that refuses to budge even after a good night's rest. There may simply be days when the fatigue is better or worse, often for no apparent reason. As a result, you may still find yourself walking around in a state of mind-numbing fatigue while trying to juggle all your responsibilities.

If that's the case, you need to take steps to minimize your fatigue, such as pacing yourself, setting priorities, and being realistic about how much you can do. But there are other things you can do to make your fatigue more bearable. While they may not make up for your lack of sleep, these measures can conserve your energy.

Essential

It's a myth that people need less sleep when they get older. In reality, older adults still need the optimal seven to nine hours of rest that younger adults do. What does happen is that sleep becomes harder to attain because of bad sleep habits that are now entrenched, greater sensitivity to noise, and illness. Older adults are also more likely to nap, which can disrupt nighttime sleep, and to suffer sleep disorders, such as restless legs syndrome.

Delegate, Delegate, Delegate

Some people have a hard time letting responsibilities go. They don't trust their spouses to clean the house the right way, their children to do chores, or their colleagues to do a good job. Now that you have fibromyalgia, you have to forget these notions and rely on the people around you for assistance. Get in the habit of handing out responsibilities to people around you and accepting that things will not necessarily be done the way you want them done.

At home, that means asking your spouse, roommate, or children to step up to the plate and do chores you normally handled. Even little kids can empty small wastebaskets, make beds, and load a dishwasher. It helps if you can make a game of it. At work, it means asking colleagues and subordinates to handle a little more on a bad day.

Some people have a hard time handing off tasks to others. You may think that you're the only one who can do the job right. If that sounds like you, practice doling out the less important tasks first, then work toward delegating more critical ones, if necessary. With practice, and as you slowly learn to let go, it will get easier.

Learn to Say No

While it might have been exciting to delve into new projects in the past, conserving your energy has now become more important. That's why you need to learn how to say no. For some people, saying no doesn't come easily. If you're one of them, try posting some stock phrases near the phone or by the computer. That way, when a request comes via telephone or e-mail, you'll be ready with a response. Good answers might be, "I'd love to help, but this is not a good time for me," or "Gee, that sounds interesting, but I'm really not the right person for it." Or if you choose to be more direct, you can simply say, "Thank you for asking. But I'm going to have to say no right now."

If saying no still doesn't come easily to you, look for other strategies that might make you less uneasy. For instance, if your boss is deluging you with work, ask him to prioritize what's most important so you know where to focus your efforts. Or if a volunteer group leader asks you to do yet another task, find out if there's another obligation that you can drop. The goal is to ensure that you don't let others impose too many responsibilities on you—responsibilities that will eventually tire you out. Remember, healthy people set healthy boundaries.

Balance Rest and Activity

In a society that puts a premium on achievement, stopping to take a rest might seem entirely counterintuitive. But for someone who has fibromyalgia, rest is critical to keeping fatigue at bay.

For fibro patients, energy is like money in your bank account. If you just spend and spend, you're going to run out. Rest, on the other hand, is like making a deposit or an investment in your well-being. For someone with fibromyalgia, it's important to make as many deposits as possible.

Balancing rest and activity doesn't mean that you should be confined to bed or that you should concede defeat. What it does mean is that you should simply stop and take a regular break—before you feel overexerted. If you're having a particularly bad time, you might need to put more emphasis on rest and less on activity. During periods of remission, you might get away with doing a little more. The key is always giving your body the opportunity to rest.

Nap, If Needed

In some cultures, an afternoon nap is a cherished part of the routine. But in our hectic lives, most people regard napping as an indulgence that disrupts progress on the to-do list. For people with fibromyalgia, however, a nap may be necessary, particularly if their sleep has been especially bad.

Alert

Resist the urge to grab a cup of coffee to keep you going. Caffeine is a stimulant that can keep you awake. But after it wears off, it leaves you even more tired than before. You should also avoid other foods and drinks that contain caffeine, such as tea, soda, energy drinks, and anything that contains chocolate.

If you do choose to nap, do it in the early afternoon. Avoid sleeping too long, since that can make it harder for you to sleep later on.

Experiment with the amount of time that works best for you. For some people, that might mean napping for just fifteen to twenty minutes, while others may be able to sleep as much as forty-five minutes.

Exhausting Emotions

The guilt. The perfectionism. The frustration. Learning to let go of some of these exhausting emotions can help rid you of fatigue as well. For instance, if you're constantly feeling the pressure to have a perfectly clean house, you are not only working toward getting it there. You are also emotionally exhausted by the impossible standards you have set.

Try to let go of feelings that tire you out by setting more realistic expectations. For instance, if you're fraught with guilt over not participating in your child's classroom because you're sick, try helping out by donating some art supplies instead. Or if you're angry over your inability to keep a clean house anymore, try to be content with just keeping one room clean.

It may not be easy if you've grown accustomed to living with these expectations all your life. But here's a paradox to consider: Perfectionism can be a flaw! To help you get over it, try talking with a good friend, a clergy person, or a therapist, any of whom might be able to help you change your perspective. Chapter 15 discusses emotional challenges in greater detail.

CHAPTER 8

The Sleep Problem

Pain is one of the leading causes of insomnia, so it should come as no surprise that people with fibromyalgia are often victims of poor sleep. In fact, getting a good night's sleep might seem like a total luxury to you, one that's become unattainable. But there are things you can do to improve your sleep and reduce your fatigue. In this chapter, we'll take a look at sleep, why yours may be troubled, and how you can get more of it.

What Is Sleep?

Sleep is a major part of health and well-being—and a big part of our lives as well. We spend a third of our lives in a state of sleep. But our modern understanding of sleep was developed only in the last century, when scientists became intrigued by the eye movements they saw in sleeping infants. Until that time, most people didn't realize the vital role that sleep plays in our health and well-being, including the way sleep actually helps improve your mental and emotional function and even has a role in the formation of memories.

Research revealed that sleep actually occurred in five distinct stages, which are divided into REM (rapid eye movement) sleep and NREM (non–rapid eye movement) sleep. NREM, the first part of the sleep cycle, breaks down into four stages that can be measured by the electrical waves seen on an electroencephalogram (EEG) machine.

In stage one, you transition from being awake to being asleep. You gradually lose awareness of your surroundings, and your breathing begins to slow. As you progress from stage one to stage two, your sleep deepens. Together, stages one and two are known as alpha sleep, named for the waves seen on an EEG.

In stages three and four, you experience your most restorative sleep. The brain waves in this stage, called delta waves, are very slow. In these stages, you are immersed in your deepest phases of sleep and least likely to be awakened. Your heartbeat and breathing become very slow and regular, and your body achieves a state of deep relaxation. It is during these two final stages that your body secretes important immune-boosting substances and growth hormone, a substance for repairing muscles. Without these two stages of sleep, you do not awaken feeling refreshed.

Throughout the night, you move gradually from each level of sleep to the next, without ever skipping over a phase. Interestingly, it's only from stage one that you move into REM sleep, the stage of sleep in which dreams occur. In REM, your brain is also undergoing the process of storing long-term memory. Some people even notice that they experience a dreamlike state as they're falling asleep. Though most people reach REM sleep ninety minutes after they first fall asleep, the bulk of REM sleep occurs toward the end of a night's rest. The five stages of sleep continue to cycle throughout the night, with the sleeper spending a total of sixty to ninety minutes in each stage. During a typical night, a healthy person will repeat each cycle several times a night.

Now that you have fibromyalgia, sound sleep might seem like an entirely foreign concept. Whether it's the pain that causes sleep disturbance, or the sleep disturbance that is causing the pain remains uncertain. But as many as 90 percent of all people with fibromyalgia report having sleep problems.

Fibro Sleep

In people who have fibromyalgia, sleep is poor. Even patients who have little trouble falling asleep or who stay in bed an entire night can awaken feeling unrefreshed, sometimes feeling as if they didn't really sleep at all. Tests have shown that the reason for poor sleep can be traced to a malfunction in the sleep process at stages three and four—essential stages for secreting important hormones and repairing body tissue. In fact, many FMS sufferers do not ever fully achieve stage three or four sleep because of a condition called alpha-EEG anomaly, in which regular bursts of alpha (waking) brain wave activity intrude just as they're going into deep sleep. As a result, even when they're "sleeping," some people with fibromyalgia may not ever be fully asleep.

L. Essential

If your nighttime sleep problems are accompanied by heartburn, you may be experiencing GERD (gastroesophageal reflux disease), a common gastrointestinal illness that affects about 7 percent of all U.S. adults. The backflow of acid from the stomach into the esophagus can cause irritation of the esophageal lining, belching, difficulty swallowing, and coughing. Left untreated, GERD can lead to Barrett's esophagus, which can become cancerous.

Some people notice that their sleep problems change. You may have nights when you can't sleep at all. On other nights, you may not drift off until 3 A.M. Still other nights, you may fall asleep quickly only to awaken abruptly and be unable to return to sleep.

If your problems are mild, you may experience mild fatigue. But many people with fibromyalgia experience a type of crushing fatigue that makes even the simplest task seem insurmountable.

Several aspects of fibromyalgia conspire to make sleep a challenge. When you're in the throes of chronic pain, it's hard to get comfortable and relax. You may also be experiencing tremendous stress and anxiety from having a chronic health problem. In addition, you may be suffering from depression, which can interfere with your ability to sleep.

Other Sleep Problems

People with fibromyalgia are also more likely to have other sleep conditions that prevent them from getting a good night's rest. In addition to alpha-delta sleep anomaly, people who have fibro may experience restless legs syndrome (RLS), periodic limb movements during sleep, and sleep apnea. Many grind their teeth during sleep, a condition known as bruxism that is associated with temporomandibular joint disorder and wearing down of the teeth.

RLS

People who have RLS often describe a creepy crawly sensation in their legs that usually occurs at night. Approximately 20 to 40 percent of people with FMS suffer from this neurological condition, which afflicts about 8 percent of all adults in the United States.

The condition makes your legs feel twitchy, uneasy, and tingly. These sensations cause an overwhelming urge to move the legs. Often, the only way to get relief from these uncomfortable sensations is to get up and move. Some people can find relief from RLS by taking a walk, stretching, taking a hot or cold bath, or massaging the affected leg. Sometimes, practicing relaxation techniques such as meditation or yoga can help. Reducing stress and giving up cigarettes and caffeine might also help. But others may need medications to help reduce or relieve their symptoms.

Alert

Next time you're feeling drowsy on the road, pull over for a fifteen- to forty-five-minute nap. According to the National Sleep Foundation, opening the window, turning up the music, and blasting the air conditioning are ineffective ways of keeping you awake behind the wheel. Caffeinated beverages like coffee can help for a little while, but the caffeine doesn't kick in for about thirty minutes.

Periodic Limb Movements During Sleep (PLMS)

About 80 percent of people with RLS also have periodic leg movements during sleep (PLMS). PLMS is characterized by herky-jerky maneuvers of the legs and feet that occur as frequently as every half a second but usually every twenty to forty seconds. The motion is involuntary and may sometimes be strong enough to hurt someone sleeping beside you. They may also vary a great deal; some people have small imperceptible movement, while others may be flailing. In rare cases, the movements involve the arms. Either way, the involuntary nighttime motions inhibit sound sleep and leave its sufferers exhausted. Most people who have PLMS are aged 65 or older. The condition occurs equally in men and women. Although the cause of PLMS remains a mystery, experts believe it may involve the nervous system.

PLMS is generally not considered a serious medical problem. But the constant movement can disturb sleep and exacerbate fatigue. That's because every time you move, you go from a deeper state of sleep to a lighter one, making it hard for you to get the restorative sleep you need in the deeper stages. As a result, getting treatment for RLS and PLMS is important for fibromyalgia patients.

Sleep Apnea

Approximately 18 million people in the United States have sleep apnea, a potentially serious sleep disorder that occurs when you actually stop breathing for ten to thirty seconds at a time while you're asleep. These brief spells can occur as many as 400 times a night, and they prevent a good night's rest. During sleep, the person with sleep apnea may frequently snore, pause, and gasp. Some people are unaware they have sleep apnea until a family member alerts them to their loud snoring.

Most people with sleep apnea have obstructive apnea, which means something is blocking the windpipe, or trachea, which brings air into your body. Efforts to breathe are blocked by the tongue, tonsils, or uvula, the little piece of flesh that hangs in the back of your throat. Excess fatty tissue in the throat or even relaxed throat muscles can cause obstructive sleep apnea, too. Sleep apnea is more common in men with fibromyalgia than it is in women. The majority of people who have it are overweight.

In some people, sleep apnea can cause depression, memory problems, and difficulties concentrating. It may also contribute to high blood pressure, heart failure, stroke, and heart attack. In addition, sleep apnea can lead to a serious heart problem called cardiomyopathy, which is diffuse damage to the heart muscle. When you stop breathing as you sleep, the oxygen levels in your blood drop. Your heart can't stop beating, so it continues to work with less oxygen than it needs. The low oxygen levels can damage the heart tissue. If not caught early, this condition can be fatal.

The most common way to treat sleep apnea is through weight reduction. But there are also devices that can be used to improve breathing. Continuous positive airway pressure treatment, for instance, involves an apparatus that uses a nasal mask to blow air from a fan into the nostrils to keep the airway open.

Bruxism

The nighttime result of daytime stress can sometimes result in bruxism, the clenching or grinding of teeth. Bruxism can often lead to temporomandibular joint disorder. Some people who clamp their teeth together also grind their teeth, in a sideways or back-and-forth movement.

As you might imagine, doing this to your teeth every night can wear down the enamel on your teeth and can lead to jaw pain, headaches, and ear problems. It can also worsen existing dental problems. The nightly grinding may go unnoticed until the dentist detects unusual wear on the surface of the teeth. Usually, bruxism is a result of too much stress.

Treating bruxism requires a multipronged approach that involves reducing the clenching, limiting damage to the teeth, and minimizing the pain. Making an effort to relax your jaw muscles throughout the day can help reduce the clenching. You should also try to reduce stress by doing relaxation exercises such as meditation. In addition, invest in a night guard that will help prevent damage to your teeth.

To eliminate pain, you can try applying ice or heat to a sore jaw. You may also find relief with help from a massage therapist.

The Insomnia Battle

You know the routine. Night after night, you lie there awake, tossing and turning, waiting for sweet slumber to set in. The clock inches ahead, and you feel the frustration rising as you brace yourself for another sleepless night—and another exhausting day. Sound familiar? If you suffer from insomnia, you're in good company. According to a 2002 poll by the National Sleep Foundation, 58 percent of all U.S. adults experience insomnia at least a few nights a week. But insomnia isn't just about difficulty falling asleep. People who can't maintain sleep or who awaken too early every morning are also suffering from insomnia. The end result is always the same: You go through your days feeling tired and irritable.

Question

Why not test for substance P?
Several studies have determined that people with fibromyalgia average three times more substance P in their spinal fluid than healthy people. But it's hardly a conclusive diagnostic tool. Some fibro patients have normal levels, and elevated levels are also present in people who have osteoarthritis and chronic back pain. Getting tested for substance P also isn't easy and requires a spinal tap.

It's not uncommon for people who have fibromyalgia to have insomnia. The sleeplessness is typically the result of chronic pain. The pain, in turn, creates frequent intrusions by overactive alpha waves that prevent you from sleeping. As a result, you become even more sensitive to pain, and a vicious cycle of pain and sleeplessness results. On top of that, people with fibromyalgia are often under tremendous stress. Even healthy people are vulnerable to sleep loss when they're stressed out and anxious. Compounding the stress is the inability to sleep, which creates yet another vicious cycle of sleeplessness.

Sleep Solutions

Finding a way to improve the quality of your sleep is important, so if you're having problems getting enough rest, you should discuss it with your doctor. Your doctor may prescribe a sleep medication. In the meantime, you can take steps to improve your sleep hygiene. Different strategies will work for different people, and it may take some trial and error to figure out what helps you sleep. Take Jean, who devised her own sleep routine that involved several changes.

Jean has always wrestled with insomnia. But rather than taking medications, she chose to eat foods that helped promote sleep. An hour before bed, she often drinks warm milk with honey, or has oatmeal with warm milk. At the same time, she avoids high-protein foods, spicy foods, and decaffeinated coffee, which can all keep her awake. As a result, she's been waking less often and sleeping better.

Other people can achieve better sleep by making simple changes in their habits, schedule, and routine. Here are some suggestions from the National Sleep Foundation.

- **Keep it regular.** Get up and go to bed at the same time every day, even on weekends. Resisting the urge to sleep in on a Saturday morning will help your body establish and sustain a regular wake-sleep cycle.
- **Make your bedroom sleep-friendly.** Keep the room cool, quiet, and dark. Minimize auditory distractions by using humidifiers or fans that create white noise, which can lull some people to sleep. Use dark shades to minimize light.

- **Make it comfortable.** If your mattress is older than nine or ten years, it might be time to replace it. When you do, select one that is comfortable and supportive. Spend fifteen minutes testing it out in the store before you buy.
- **Keep the temperature just right.** Avoid making your room too warm or too cool. Experiment and find a temperature setting that doesn't bother you.
- **Use your bedroom only for sleep and sex.** Leave your work in the office and the television in the living room. Limiting activities in your bedroom will help you associate the room with sleep.
- **Exercise regularly.** Regular physical activity can promote sleep. But try to do it at least three hours before bedtime. The best time is in the late afternoon.
- **Get up if you can't sleep.** Rather than lie there, get up and do something unstimulating. Try reading a dull book, folding laundry, or watching television. When you start feeling tired, go back and try again.
- **Don't take worries to bed.** Before going to bed, write down your worries and make a to-do list for the next day. Then set them aside and focus your attention on relaxing.

Create a Relaxing Routine

Whether you read, listen to music, or soak in a tub, a restful routine can set the stage and relieve the stress and anxiety that make it harder to get to sleep. Try to do these things in low light, since bright lights can be arousing. Avoid stimulating activities before bed, such as paying bills, playing games, or solving problems.

Watch What You Eat and Drink

Most people are better off not eating in the two or three hours before bed. Limit fluids so you don't awaken at night for visits to the bathroom. Avoid caffeinated drinks and food such as coffee, tea, soda, and chocolate. Foods high in carbs can keep you awake, too.

📋 Fact

Poor sleep can take a toll on relationships. A 2005 poll by the National Sleep Foundation found that more than a third of adults with partners say their partner's sleep issues have caused some problems in the relationship. Twenty-three percent have taken to sleeping in another room or on the couch, and 7 percent use an eye mask or ear plugs to shut out the disturbance.

Avoid Alcohol and Nicotine

Both alcohol and nicotine can lead to poor sleep, especially when used close to bedtime. Although many people think of alcohol as a sedative, it actually causes nighttime awakenings and less restful sleep. When a smoker goes to sleep, her body actually goes into a state of withdrawal. Nicotine not only makes it hard to fall asleep, but it also makes it hard for you to wake up. Research suggests that smokers may also have more nightmares. Kicking the habit isn't easy. At first, it might even cause sleep problems. But over time, giving up cigarettes will improve your rest.

Make Sleep a Priority

There's no doubt that a good night's sleep is one of the cornerstones of good health, especially for someone who has fibromyalgia. A good night's rest can reduce your pain, lower your stress, and make your other symptoms less annoying.

So be on the lookout for health conditions such as restless legs syndrome or sleep apnea that may disturb sleep. If necessary, get these conditions treated. Take steps to improve your sleep hygiene, and create the environment and habits that will promote sound sleep. If all else fails, consult your physician about what else you can do. You may require medications to help you get back on track.

CHAPTER 9

Other Fibro Troubles

Pain and fatigue are tough enough by themselves, but many fibromyalgia sufferers also endure other symptoms. You may have persistent headaches, stomach troubles, and jaw pain. You may suffer depression and cognitive problems that make it hard to do your job. In this chapter, we offer you a head-to-toe guide on other conditions that often occur with fibromyalgia. Hopefully, by understanding them, you'll be better able to cope with these conditions and better equipped to treat them.

The Brain

Headaches. Memory problems. Depression. At the root of all these symptoms is the brain, your body's command central for all bodily functions. It should come as no surprise that fibromyalgia takes a profound toll on your head. Whether it's cognitive problems or persistent headaches, your brain may experience problems related to fibromyalgia.

Fibro Fog

Almost everyone has flashes of confusion. Misplacing that all-important car key. Going into a room for a reason that escapes you. Losing your car in a parking lot with no memory of where you left it. But for some people who have fibromyalgia, this confusion leads to a condition affectionately known as fibro fog. With fibro fog, you have difficulty remembering familiar facts, focusing, and concentrating. Fibro fog can make it hard for you to do your job, perform daily tasks, and follow simple directions.

Studies show that fibromyalgia patients who report poor memory demonstrate it on tests that measure recall. In fact, one study has shown that people with FMS do no better on cognitive performance tests than people who are twenty years older—though they perform just as well as healthy peers on tests that measured speed of cognition.

Chances are that poor sleep contributes to fibro fog. Experts suspect that people with fibromyalgia may also be getting less oxygen into their brains. Other possible causes include depression, a malfunction in the central nervous system, and certain medications. For some people, like Nancy, these cognitive challenges are the most frustrating symptoms of all.

> Nancy describes fibro fog as "swimming through Jell-O." In the last two years, fibro fog has been her most challenging symptom. When she's in the throes of it, Nancy cannot recall simple words. She cannot remember her best friend's name, even when she's looking at her. Making decisions becomes impossible because she cannot even put two and two together. She tries to keep lists to help her remember. But some days Nancy can't even remember where she put the list. The severity of her cognitive problems, she says, is directly correlated to her pain and fatigue. The worse her pain and fatigue, the worse her fibro fog is.

Getting a handle on fibro fog requires minimizing your pain and fatigue. That means trying to get a good night's sleep and reducing stress. If your memory problems are severe, however, you may need professional help. When you're in the throes of a bout of fibro fog, try the following tips:

- Make lists for everything. Whether it's a grocery list or a to-do list, jot down specifically what you need.
- Keep your lists in places you can remember.
- If necessary, take notes when meeting with people, such as your boss or your doctor.
- Use strategically placed sticky notes to help you remember.

Depression

It's easy to understand why a chronic illness like fibromyalgia can bring on depression. The constant pain, lack of sleep, and persistent fatigue can devastate even the most cheerful people. As a result, you may start to feel hopeless and sad, which can spiral into full-blown depression.

Although everyone gets sad from time to time, serious depression is a mental illness that can cause tremendous pain and suffering. According to the National Institutes of Mental Health, almost 19 million people suffer from a depressive illness in a given year, or 9.5 percent of the population. Women are affected twice as often as men.

Of course, it's entirely normal to feel sad about having fibromyalgia, just as it is when you lose your job, a loved one, or a pet. The grief is a reaction to a downturn in your life. But distinguishing depression from the blues isn't easy. Many of its signs and symptoms are easily blamed on stress, fatigue, and a hectic lifestyle. As a result, depression often goes unrecognized. Left untreated, depression can worsen your fibromyalgia, weaken your immune system, and destroy your quality of life.

The key is the intensity of the symptoms and the duration of the problem. Depression is also accompanied by a pervasive sense of helplessness and hopelessness. When you lose interest in activities you normally enjoy, it might signal that something is wrong, especially if the lethargy lasts for more than two weeks. And if you're feeling so bad about yourself that you can no longer get along with loved ones or colleagues, then your depression is starting to interfere with your functioning. Here's a checklist to help you determine whether you have depression. If any of these problems persists for two weeks or more, you may need professional attention:

- Frequent sadness, often accompanied by crying
- Feelings of hopelessness, helplessness, and worthlessness
- Loss of interest in things that normally bring you pleasure
- Irritability
- Difficulties getting along at work and at home

- Trouble concentrating and forgetfulness
- Unexplained physical complaints, such as headaches and stomach pains
- Changes in appetite
- Changes in the amount of sleep you get
- Thoughts of suicide

Depression can be hazardous and make it harder for you to take care of yourself. Don't take depression lightly—it is the most serious complication of fibromyalgia because it can create suicidal thoughts. Call your physician immediately if you or those who care about you suspect you're depressed.

Headaches

Everyone suffers a headache at one time or another. A long commute, an argument with your teenaged son, and even too much coffee can trigger a headache. But people who have fibromyalgia may be more vulnerable to headaches than the average person. Experts estimate that approximately 50 percent of people with fibromyalgia suffer from recurrent migraine or tension headaches. Chronic headaches of any kind can be disruptive and interfere with daily activities.

Causes and Effects

Numerous factors can trigger a headache. Certain foods, odors, your period, and the weather can all set off that throbbing ache. So can difficult emotions, such as stress, depression, anxiety, disappointment, and frustration. Myofascial trigger points are another activator, as are certain habits, including too much time in front of a computer, sleeping in an awkward position, and consuming too much caffeine.

Some headaches are more debilitating than others. Many people with fibromyalgia suffer from migraine headaches, an intense throbbing pain that often occurs on one side of the head. Migraines can also bring on muscle tenderness, fatigue, mood changes, and nausea and vomiting. The severity of a migraine varies, as does the event that triggers it. Some people become sensitive to light and sound when they're having a migraine.

Ĺ. Essential

A survey by the National Headache Foundation found that most migraine sufferers don't take advantage of preventive strategies to relieve their pain. The poll found that only 20 percent of migraine sufferers use preventive medications. Experts believe that using therapies to prevent migraines can reduce their incidence by as much as 80 percent.

Some experts believe that migraines and fibromyalgia belong to a group of disorders involving a malfunction of the brain's pain center. The two conditions share similar symptoms, including depression, anxiety, and sleep disturbance. Often, if a treatment relieves migraines, you may find that it improves fibromyalgia symptoms, too.

Of course, not all fibromyalgia sufferers have migraines. Some simply have tension headaches, which are more common. Tension headaches are generally the result of tight muscles in the neck or shoulders, which may come from holding your head in one position for too long. Unlike migraines, tension headaches are constant, not throbbing. They generally don't make you sensitive to light or noise.

Treating Headaches

Occasional tension headaches may be relieved with an over-the-counter remedy such as acetaminophen or ibuprofen. But if your headaches are painful and become chronic, you should talk to your doctor about more targeted treatment options. People who experience migraines have several medication options. You can take drugs that prevent migraines, relieve the pain of an attack, or sometimes, both. Drugs that provide relief include antidepressants, antiepileptics, pain medications, and triptans, a newer class of medications that narrow blood vessels and balance brain chemicals. Some doctors may prescribe a combination of caffeine and ergotamine, a drug that reduces pain by narrowing the blood vessels. Some people may find relief through alternative methods such as biofeedback.

But you can also practice some self-care strategies. Be on the lookout for events that trigger a headache and try to avoid them. Eat a healthy diet, quit smoking, and reduce your alcohol intake. During a headache, you can try to self-treat with these suggestions from the National Headache Foundation:

- Try breathing deeply and slowly from your diaphragm.
- Take a warm shower or bath.
- Apply ice or heat to the part of your head that hurts.
- Consider massage, which helps you relax and relieves stress.

Most of us reach for an analgesic like acetaminophen or aspirin at the first sign of a headache. But used daily, or almost daily, analgesics can make matters worse by causing rebound headaches. Quitting analgesics after extended use may only worsen the symptoms for three to five days. After that, you should notice an improvement. So while analgesics may temporarily reduce headache pain, be wary of overuse.

The Eyes and Mouth

Everyone knows the dry, gritty feeling in their eyes that sometimes comes with allergy season, a smoky bar, or contact lenses that are overdue for replacement. And you probably know the feeling of dryness in your mouth that comes from a lack of water. But if you have fibromyalgia, dryness of the eyes and mouth may occur for no apparent reason.

If this dryness of the eyes and mouth becomes a major problem, it is known as sicca syndrome. It's not uncommon for people who have fibromyalgia to lose moisture in their mucous membranes. In the mouth, the dryness may be compounded by a reduction of saliva produced by the salivary glands. In most cases, the eyes are more vulnerable than the mouth.

Although uncomfortable, dry eyes—which may also burn, sting, or appear red—are often treatable with over-the-counter lubricating drops or artificial tears. According to Devin Starlanyl in her book, *Fibromyalgia and Chronic Myofascial Pain,* using drops that can be stored in the refrigerator can provide added relief, since the cold naturally helps constrict swollen blood vessels in the eye. To treat dry mouth, talk to your physician. You might also try sipping water regularly, sucking on a sugar-free hard candy, or chewing sugar-free gum.

Vision Problems

In some people, fibromyalgia can take a toll on eyesight, especially if you have headaches. You may notice that you have difficulty focusing on objects that are close up. At night, sensitivity to light might make it hard for you to drive in the face of oncoming traffic.

If you have vision problems, talk to your doctor. You may also need to see an ophthalmologist or optometrist, eye-care specialists who can help correct poor vision. It can help to wear polarized sunglasses, which can reduce glare.

Jaw and Dental Problems

In the middle of the night, when you think you've escaped your stressors with some much-needed zzzzs, your teeth may become the unwitting victim of lingering stress. As a result, you may grind, gnash, and clench your teeth. The result of all this nighttime grinding—also called bruxism—can be temporomandibular joint disorder, or TMJ. TMJ affects the joint that connects the upper jaw to the lower jaw, which you have on both sides of your face. It also affects the ligaments and muscles surrounding the joint.

TMJ is common in people who have fibromyalgia, especially women. But it can also occur with aging, injury, and even excessive gum chewing. People who have TMJ typically experience stiffness, headaches, and ear pain. They may hear grinding and clicking noises in their jaw, and the jaws may even lock. Some people with TMJ develop dental problems, too, as the grinding of teeth slowly erodes the enamel.

In people who have fibromyalgia, TMJ is often related to stress. That's why treatment usually involves relaxation exercises, facial massage, and the application of hot, moist packs to the jaw at bedtime. You may also consider talking to an occupational therapist, who can suggest new ways of chewing and eating that can ease your jaw pain. Myofascial therapy is often helpful, too. If TMJ becomes severe, surgery may be necessary.

Fact

A mouth guard is often the best way to protect your teeth from the damage of grinding. These are available through your dentist. Some people may find that the mouth guards sold in sporting good stores do the trick—and much less expensively, too.

Tummy Troubles

Estimates show that 50 to 75 percent of people with fibromyalgia suffer from irritable bowel syndrome (IBS). IBS is a chronic gastrointestinal condition characterized by cramps, abdominal pain, bloating, constipation, and diarrhea. No one knows exactly what causes IBS, but we do know it involves a malfunction of the large intestine. Nerves and muscles in the large intestine may contract too much or be overly sensitive to certain stimuli such as foods or stress. Other triggers include eating a large meal, menstruation, and sensitivities to certain foods and medication. As a result, stool may pass too quickly or slowly through the intestines, resulting in diarrhea or constipation. Sometimes, you may feel an overwhelming urge to have a bowel movement only to find that you can't.

IBS can be a major nuisance that disrupts everyday activities such as working, socializing with friends, and traveling. Albeit annoying, the condition does not cause permanent damage to the intestines and does not lead to serious diseases such as cancer.

Treating IBS often involves altering your diet to include more high-fiber foods, such as whole-grain pasta and breads. At the same time, you may need to cut back on fried foods, high-fat foods, coffee, caffeine, and alcohol. Certain sugars can trigger IBS in some people as well. In others, certain vegetables, such as broccoli, cabbage, and beans, may cause gassiness. Still others may need to avoid gluten, a chemical found in many grains. Keeping a food diary and recording your symptoms can help you pin down the foods that irritate you.

Taking steps to alleviate stress is almost always a part of treating IBS. Some people get relief with meditation, biofeedback, and hypnosis. In some cases, you may need to treat the symptoms. Some people treat constipation with laxatives, while those with loose stools may require antidiarrhea medications. All laxatives should be used only for the short-term since they can be habit-forming. Your doctor may prescribe a medication specifically approved for IBS if your symptoms are severe and don't respond to dietary changes and stress management. Psyllium and enteric-coated peppermint oil are often helpful, too. In some cases, an antidepressant can help. For more information about IBS, check out the Web site for the Irritable Bowel Syndrome Self-Help and Support Group, at *www.ibsgroup.org*.

Question

Why would you give an antidepressant for IBS?
The brain isn't the only organ that houses neurotransmitters like serotonin. The intestines do, too. In fact, some people consider the gut the "other brain" and call it the enteric nervous system. IBS is thought to be a disruption of serotonin signals between the gut and the brain. Antidepressants work by restoring balance to serotonin levels in the intestines as well as the brain.

Urinary Troubles

People who have fibromyalgia are vulnerable to interstitial cystitis (IC), a chronic and painful inflammation of the bladder. Like fibromyalgia and IBS, the cause of IC is a mystery. People who have IC typically experience an increased need to urinate. In some people, it may feel urgent. If you have a severe case, you may wind up urinating as many as sixty times a day. It can also cause pain in the pelvic region, especially during sexual intercourse and/or menstruation.

Treating IC often requires a great deal of trial and error. The only medication currently approved by the FDA for use in treating IC is pentosan polysulfate (Elmiron), which can relieve bladder discomfort and pain by preventing irritation of the bladder lining. Certain tricyclic antidepressants, anti-inflammatories, antispasmodics, antihistamines, and muscle relaxants can also provide relief. Some patients may be treated with bladder instillation, which involves pouring medications into the bladder. In rare cases, surgery may be done, though it's often not successful.

You can also take self-help measures to alleviate your symptoms. Eliminating highly acidic or spicy foods can reduce the symptoms, as can giving up cigarettes, caffeine, and alcohol. You might also consider trying stress reduction strategies, such as exercise and meditation. For more information about IC, check out the Interstitial Cystitis Association Web site at *www.ichelp.com*.

Menstrual Problems

If you had bad menstrual problems in the past, chances are that they got worse when you developed fibromyalgia. This is especially true during a flare-up. You may experience more cramps, irregular blood flow, blood clots, or greater-than-normal blood flow. And if you suffer from PMS, those symptoms may worsen as well.

If your periods have become intolerable, talk to your primary doctor or OB-GYN and get help. Getting enough sleep, conserving your energy levels, and eating a healthy diet can help minimize menstrual symptoms, too. And anti-inflammatories or antidepressants may be beneficial in severe cases.

Vaginal Pain

For some women with fibromyalgia, pain strikes the vulva and produces a condition known as vulvodynia. The vulva is the external female genitalia, which includes the tissue at the base of your abdomen, the labia, the clitoris, and the opening of your vagina. Vulvodynia may cause burning, stinging, rawness, and overall soreness. You may also feel itchy and uncomfortable. Upon examination, however, there is no apparent problem. Still, the painful sensations continue—sometimes occurring intermittently, other times lasting for longer periods. Vulvodynia can make it impossible for you to have sex, which can affect your relationship. It can also bring on depression, especially if the suffering begins to interfere with daily functioning.

 Fact

A study by researchers at the University of Michigan found that women with vulvodynia don't just have more pain in their genitals. They also experience more pain in the shin, thumbnail, and the deltoid muscle in the shoulder. The findings lend further proof to the idea that vulvodynia is part of a systemic problem with pain, not a sexual disorder or psychosomatic problem.

Treating vulvodynia may involve a tricyclic antidepressant, an anticonvulsant, or an antihistamine, which targets itchiness. Creams that contain estrogen or cortisone can sometimes provide relief, too. In some women, applying an anesthesia cream such as lidocaine can ease the pain. Sometimes a cold compress can help as well. Physical treatments such as myofascial therapy to the pelvic muscles can often be very effective, too. In some cases, you may be able to take steps to prevent vulvodynia or at least lessen the painful symptoms. Avoid soaps, hygiene products, and tight-fitting undergarments. In some cases, exercise can help relieve discomfort.

Problems All Over

As you can see, fibromyalgia can make its presence known in some specific parts of your body. But some problems seem to crop up everywhere and anywhere, affecting your entire sense of well-being. Like most fibro problems, these symptoms may come and go, and they may not always strike the same area. But they can be extremely disturbing nonetheless. In this section, we'll take a look at fibro troubles that can affect you all over.

Numbness or Tingling

Almost a third of fibromyalgia patients will experience numbness or tingling at some point. Some may complain of feeling numb or tingly all over. Others experience a loss of sensation in a limb. Often, there is no pattern to the numbness. These feelings may occur intermittently anywhere on the body, and they may change from day to day.

 Alert

Fibro sufferers are vulnerable to carpal tunnel syndrome, a compression of the median nerve in the wrist that can cause swelling in the wrist and tingling in the fingers. Be wary of surgery to treat carpal tunnel, though. Research suggests that people with fibromyalgia have less success with surgery. Lifestyle change, wrist supports, physical therapy, or possibly cortisone injections should be tried first.

Numbness and tingling are often the result of an injury to a nerve that supplies blood to the affected body part. It may also be caused by something as simple as staying in the same position for too long. An imbalance of electrolytes or minerals in your body can also cause numbness, as can certain medications or medical conditions such as diabetes, migraine headaches, or hypothyroidism.

Getting rid of the numbness or tingling often means resolving another condition. For instance, if you're suffering an electrolyte imbalance, you may need to eat more of the missing electrolyte. But in some people with fibromyalgia, the numbness and tingling may exist without any apparent cause. Consider Paula, who first experienced numbness after a car accident two years ago that triggered the onset of fibromyalgia.

> These days, Paula sometimes wakes up feeling numb for no apparent reason. To combat the numbness, she loosens her muscles with stretching exercises. She also applies heat packs on her muscles to relax them. Sometimes, she gets relief with a hot bath and shower. Doctors, she says, frequently ask about numbness, but they often attribute it to other ailments. But Paula thinks it's mostly the result of her fibromyalgia.

If you do experience numbness or tingling, discuss it with your doctor.

Oversensitivity—To Everything

A whiff of new carpeting sets off uncontrolled sneezing. Sleeping on sheets washed in a certain laundry detergent makes you itch. Walking past a fish market sets off a bout of severe nausea. If you've become hypersensitive to the smells, noises, and chemicals around you, you may have multiple chemical sensitivities (MCS) or idiopathic environmental intolerances (IEI).

Estimates vary, but as many as 50 percent of people with fibromyalgia suffer from IEI. Often, people with IEI have problems eating certain foods as well. They're often unable to tolerate alcohol, cleaning products, cigarette smoke, pollutants, pesticides, gas, paint, noise, bright lights, and perfumes. Even at low levels, these substances can trigger physical symptoms ranging from ones that resemble an allergic reaction to nausea, vomiting, headaches, and dizziness.

Some experts don't believe that IEI is real. In fact, several medical organizations—including the American Academy of Allergies Asthma & Immunology and the American Medical Association—have pointed to a lack of scientific evidence that the condition exists. It also doesn't help that there is no way to firmly diagnose whether a patient has IEI.

But that doesn't mean the suffering is any less real for the sensitive. The only way to deal with IEI right now is to pinpoint the offending substance and to try and avoid it. Although avoiding all chemicals in this day and age is virtually impossible, you can make choices about the cleaning products you use, the perfumes and hygiene products you wear, and the scents that fill your home. Surround yourself with natural fabrics instead of synthetic ones, which always contain chemicals. And do your best to avoid environments where you may come in contact with offending substances, such as candle stores and carpet warehouses.

L. Essential

Buildings have been known to make people sick. The condition is called sick building syndrome and occurs when occupants suffer health problems with no apparent illness or cause. Symptoms include headache; irritation of the eyes, nose, or throat; dry cough; dry, itchy skin; dizziness and nausea; and sensitivity to odors. Possible causes include chemicals, poor ventilation, and mold and bacteria. Relief? Treat the mold or leave the building.

Candida (Yeast) Hypersensitivity

Everyone has candida albicans living in their bodies. This exotic-sounding yeast lurks in your gastrointestinal tract, mouth, and vagina, and even parts of your skin. In healthy amounts, the yeast does no harm whatsoever. But when an imbalance occurs, and the yeast in your intestine grows unchecked, it may activate your immune system to cause a condition known as candida hypersensitivity syndrome.

Ordinary yeast infections can occur in people who take antibiotics or immune suppressant medications, which can destroy the bacteria that normally kill the fungi. Pregnant women and people with diabetes are also vulnerable to candidiasis. But in people who have fibromyalgia, a yeast infection can become a chronic problem.

Fact

Exactly what chemicals are given off by yeast to cause fibro symptoms is a mystery. We do know that yeasts can release dozens of chemicals that can be toxic to our bodies. When our bodies absorb these substances, it interferes with thyroid, metabolism, or nervous system function, which then leads to fibromyalgia symptoms.

Not everyone with fibro develops a yeast problem, but some experts believe that yeast overgrowth is a primary cause of fibromyalgia. In fact, many patients who are treated for candida hypersensitivity experience at least some improvement in their symptoms, which lends proof to this theory. Yeast overgrowth may also be involved in other chronic ailments that seem to have no explanation such as irritable bowel syndrome, interstitial cystititis, and chronic fatigue syndrome.

If you suspect you have a yeast problem, ask your doctor for a candida test (which may be as simple as a questionnaire). Treatment should be a three-pronged approach that involves dietary strategies, medication, and acidophilus supplements. Start by reducing your carbohydrates, especially the simple ones, such as cookies, cakes, and other products that contain refined sugar. By eating fewer carbs, you starve the yeast and keep it from proliferating.

Next, ask your doctor for an antifungal medication. Since different strains of candida respond to different medications, it's important to have a stool test to grow out the yeast and test it against various anti-candida drugs. Finally, take a supplement that contains lactobacillus acidophilus, a friendly bacteria that helps inhibit yeast growth and restore balance to your body. After six months, you'll have significantly less yeast in your body. Your immune system will stop attacking the yeast overgrowth, so it can get back to the work of defending you against other infections that might aggravate your fibromyalgia.

Dizziness

Some people who have fibromyalgia experience vertigo. Simply looking at a striped pattern, driving, or reading can trigger the dizziness. These spells may result from a defect in the ability of your eye muscles to track things, or tender points in your head or neck. In some cases, the dizziness may be associated with a condition known as neurally mediated hypotension, a drop in blood pressure that results from standing up and that can produce lightheadedness.

Dizziness often stems from other problems, such as headaches, fibro fog, and fatigue. Treating some of the other problems can help relieve your dizzy spells. But talk to your physician if you are experiencing dizziness.

Raynaud's Phenomenon

While it's normal for blood vessels to constrict when they're exposed to the cold—your body is trying to preserve heat—people who have Raynaud's are extra sensitive to changes in temperatures. They may even have an attack when temperatures don't change.

During a Raynaud's attack, the blood vessels undergo vasospasms that reduce circulation to the extremities, causing fingers, toes, and even the tips of your nose or ears to turn white. When they recover, the extremities turn red, hurt, and tingle. In the meantime, you may feel abnormally cold, so that while others are perfectly comfortable in T-shirts, you may be shivering with a jacket on.

The cold isn't the only thing that can set off an attack. Stress, cigarette smoking, and even typing can set off a Raynaud's attack. Severe Raynaud's can damage the tissues of your fingers and toes and may require blood-thinning medications. But averting an attack with gloves and warm clothes is often your best defense.

CHAPTER 10

Medications That Can Help

As you know, getting relief from fibromyalgia isn't easy. Eventually, you may need medications to help you get your sleep, ease your pain, and relieve your depression. You may need drugs for some of your other symptoms, too. Knowing the medications, how they work, and their possible side effects can help you determine the drugs you need—and the ones to avoid. In this chapter, we'll take a look at your drug options.

Pain Relief

At this time, there are no drugs approved to specifically treat fibromyalgia. Rather, doctors frequently—and legally—prescribe medications approved for other illnesses to treat symptoms of different conditions. The practice is known as off-label use. That's why many of the drugs you'll read about in this chapter were originally approved to treat other conditions. But rest assured, many of these therapies have been successful in treating fibro symptoms in other people. Even better, some of them work on several symptoms at once.

Antidepressants

You go to your doctor complaining of pain and fatigue. He prescribes you an antidepressant. If you think your doctor has you pegged as someone who's simply depressed, think again. Antidepressants are one of the most commonly prescribed medications for the treatment of fibromyalgia because they can actually work on several fronts—to treat pain, improve sleep, and reduce your other symptoms, including depression. They are probably the most effective medications for long-term treatment of anxiety, too. They can even work on other symptoms such as irritable bowel syndrome and interstitial cystitis. That's because the neurotransmitters that regulate our mood—serotonin, norepinephrine, and epinephrine—are the same ones that control pain and sleep. But not all antidepressants are the same. In fact, these medications fall under several categories.

Tricyclics

Tricyclics have been prescribed to treat fibromyalgia for many years and work by restoring chemical imbalances in the brain and help induce sleep. They're also used to treat panic attacks, post-traumatic stress disorder, and obsessive-compulsive disorder. Drugs in this category include amitriptyline (Elavil), clomipramine (Anafril), imipramine pamoate (Tofranil PM), desipramine (Norpramin), and nortriptyline (Aventyl). Many people can't tolerate tricyclics because of the high incidence of side effects, including dry mouth, constipation, and blurred vision.

Selective Serotonin Reuptake Inhibitors (SSRIs)

These medications have become increasingly popular in recent years. They work by blocking the removal (and deactivation) of serotonin. Selective serotonin reuptake inhibitors (SSRIs) are the most commonly used agents for treating depression because they have fewer side effects. Common SSRIs include fluoxetine (Prozac), paroxetine (Paxil), escitalopram (Lexapro), and sertraline (Zoloft). Side effects may include headache, insomnia, and sexual problems.

Mixed Reuptake Inhibitors

These antidepressants work by balancing the amounts of other neurotransmitters besides serotonin, such as dopamine and norepinephrine. Drugs in this category include venlofaxine (Effexor), buproprion (Wellbutrin), and duloxetine (Cymbalta). Because these medications have relatively few side effects and are potent inhibitors of spinal cord pain transmission, they are among the most commonly used medications in patients with chronic pain, including fibromyalgia.

Monoamine Oxidase Inhibitors (MAOIs)

This older class of antidepressant is not commonly used for fibromyalgia and is often a treatment of last resort for depression. If ingested with certain cheeses, wines, and pickles, or medications such as decongestants, monoamine oxidase inhibitors (MAOIs) can trigger dangerously high blood pressure that leads to a stroke. Medications in this category are isoarboxazid (Marplan), phenelzine (Nardil), and tranylcyproine (Parnate). MAOIs should never be taken with other antidepressants.

 ## Alert

All antidepressants are required by law to carry a warning about increased risk for suicidal thoughts and behaviors in both children and adults. You may also become more hostile and agitated. If you do take an antidepressant, do so under your doctor's close supervision, and report any unusual thoughts or behaviors immediately.

Non-narcotic Analgesics

Analgesics are painkillers that relieve the throbbing, aching, burning, and stabbing sensations that come with fibromyalgia. They come in two basic types that vary greatly in their strength. For people who have fibromyalgia, non-narcotic analgesics can sometimes relieve mild pain. Among the most popular is acetaminophen, which is found in over 600 over-the counter medications, including cough and cold products and sinus remedies. Too much acetaminophen can damage the liver, and the toxic dose for many people is only 50 percent higher than the highest recommended dose. So be careful not to take too much, and be on the lookout for medications that already contains acetaminophen. For instance, combining a cold remedy with acetaminophen for a headache can be dangerous if the cold medicine already contains acetaminophen.

Another option is nonsteroidal anti-inflammatory drugs (NSAIDs), such as ibuprofen, naproxen, and ketoprofen. These drugs work by inhibiting substances called prostaglandins, which play a role in pain and inflammation.

For a long time, aspirin was the only NSAID available. But the debut of indomethacin in the 1950s and the subsequent NSAIDs that followed gave patients more choices and were often less irritating to the stomach. Still, these medications are not benign. Every year, many people die from intestinal bleeding due to these drugs. Today, there are twenty types of NSAIDs available, both over the counter and in stronger prescription forms. Although inflammation is not usually present in people with fibromyalgia—unless they have arthritis—NSAIDs can relieve muscle aches, headaches, and menstrual cramps often caused by fibromyalgia.

Narcotic Analgesics

You might think of narcotics as illegal street drugs, such as heroin, but there are also legal narcotics that provide pain relief. These drugs are also known as opioid analgesics, and are derived from the poppy plant. Narcotics work by acting on the central nervous system and interfering with the receptors that transmit pain.

Although frequently cited as a pain treatment, there is little evidence that the chronic use of these medications improve quality of life for fibro patients. In addition, narcotics can cause addiction and/or dependence. Many people also struggle with side effects, which include dizziness, nausea, constipation, and fatigue. Drugs in this category include hydrocodone with acetaminophen (Vicodin), tramadol (Ultram), propoxyphene (Darvocet), and oxycodone (OxyContin). As a result, narcotics are generally regarded as the choice of last resort for pain relief in fibromyalgia.

Benzodiazepines

It's not unusual for people who have fibromyalgia to feel anxious about life. They may be uneasy about performing simple tasks like cooking a meal, fretful about their shaky memories, and nervous about doing their jobs. For some people, these concerns go beyond typical day-to-day issues and become a major disruption, causing what is known as generalized anxiety disorder, or GAD. For people who have anxiety, benzodiazepines might be a treatment option. These medications help relax tense muscles and induce sleep, and have both antianxiety and mild antidepressant qualities.

For people who have restless legs syndrome, a drug in this category called clonazepam (Klonopin) can sometimes provide relief from the nighttime restlessness that disrupts sleep. Other drugs in this category include alprazolam (Xanax) and cyclobenzaprine (Flexeril).

Take benzodiazepines carefully. These medications can cause addiction and depression. They may also affect memory and cognitive function and interfere with the stress response in the HPA axis. If you decide to stop taking them, do so slowly and under your doctor's supervision. Quitting abruptly can sometimes cause a withdrawal syndrome that produces symptoms such as heart tremors and palpitations.

Also, it's important to note that SSRIs and mixed reuptake antidepressants are very effective for long-term treatment of anxiety, as is the nonbenzodiazepine buspirone (Buspar).

Muscle Relaxants

Tense muscles frequently make the symptoms of fibromyalgia even worse by exacerbating your pain and making it hard to sleep at night. That's why some doctors may prescribe muscle relaxants, usually on a temporary basis. Unfortunately, they're not very effective at relaxing muscles in people with FMS.

Muscle relaxants act on the central nervous system. Some people may feel drowsy, dizzy, confused, lightheaded, or less alert when taking these drugs. The drugs may also cause blurred vision, clumsiness, or unsteadiness. Because of their sedating properties, these meds are occasionally used as sleeping agents, but in some people, they may cause insomnia. Drugs in this category include cyclobenzaprine (Flexeril), orphenadrine (Norflex), and carisoprodol (Soma). Some muscle relaxants, such as tizinidine (Zanaflex) and baclofen (Lioresal), also relieve muscle spasms.

 Alert

It's best to stay off the road the first time you take a medication. Some drugs can cause excessive drowsiness that can make driving a serious hazard. So try to time the medication to a period when you're going to be home, where you can safely monitor side effects.

Anticonvulsants

These medications are generally used to treat epilepsy and neuropathic pain—pain caused by irritation of the nerves themselves—and can also relieve pain in fibromyalgia sufferers. They work by reducing irritability of the nerve cell membrane, including that of pain nerves. They're especially effective when the pain is a burning sensation. Medicines in this category include gabapentin (Neurontin), pregabalin (Lyrica), and divalproex (Depakote). Besides relieving pain, these drugs can also improve sleep and symptoms of depression. Side effects include dizziness, drowsiness, and blurred vision.

Topical Creams

Some people have found relief with over-the-counter creams that contain capsaicin, the same substance in a hot chili pepper, or sport creams, which contain aspirin derivatives that stimulate the skin and help block pain. One prescription topical that is generating a lot of interest contains lidocaine, a numbing agent. Although originally touted as ointments for arthritis, these creams have been found to provide temporary relief for FMS sufferers.

Injections

Getting a shot of anesthetic can sometimes provide temporary relief from fibro pain, especially if the pain is localized. Most of these injections use 1 to 2 percent lidocaine, a local anesthesia.

In recent years, some patients have had success with injections of Botox, the same botulinum toxin that has been used to eliminate wrinkles in aging skin. In small quantities, Botox works by paralyzing the muscles that are causing the painful spasms. Relief from a Botox injection can last up to three or four months, by some accounts. If you do decide to try injections, make sure to find a skilled practitioner who can do them safely.

Combining Medications

Not surprisingly, perhaps, one medication for fibromyalgia often isn't enough. Some people get relief by taking medications in combination. For instance, research has shown that a combination of amitriptyline and fluoxetine results in greater improvements in fibromyalgia symptoms than either drug alone. An experienced and knowledgeable physician can work with you to develop a program specifically designed to meet your unique needs.

 Alert

If you overdose on a tricyclic antidepressant such as Elavil, head to the emergency room immediately. An overdose of a tricyclic can cause dangerous heart rhythms that can be fatal. That's one reason why the SSRIs have surpassed the tricyclics in popularity for the treatment of depression.

Unfortunately, these medications all have potential side effects, and the combination of medications can make side effects more likely. Given how sensitive fibro patients are to drugs (and particularly to side effects), it's very important for you and your doctor to communicate closely while you're being started on new medications. Don't change your use of the medication (or stop it) unless you consult with your doctor. Some meds have the potential for complications if they're stopped too quickly. Only by working closely with your doctor will you be able to pin down the right mix that is both safe and effective.

Sleep Remedies

Few things are more frustrating than the inability to get a good night's rest, especially when the sleeplessness occurs night after night, week after week. Given how poorly fibro patients sleep, it's not a surprise that many require help from medications. Sedating antidepressants are often the first approach, since they are nonaddictive and increase deep sleep. This group includes trazodone (Desyrel), amitriptyline (Elavil), nortriptyline (Pamelor), and mirtazapine (Remeron).

Though benzodiazepines such as clonazepam (Klonopin) or alprazolam (Xanax) are sometimes used, they don't provide good quality sleep, since they increase only the light stages of sleep. Newer sleep agents such as zolpidem (Ambien), zaleplon (Sonata), and eszopiclone (Lunesta) are a better choice, since they provide a better balance of deep and light sleep. Over-the-counter medications such as diphenhydramine (Benadryl or Sominex) are generally less effective in people with fibromyalgia. They can put you to sleep, but the sleep is often of poor quality. The drugs also tend to lose their effect with repeated use.

Stimulants

While the use of stimulants for fibromyalgia is avoided whenever possible, they may be used in dire situations, for instance, when school or job performance is deteriorating severely. One stimulant, modafinil (Provigil), has significantly fewer side effects than most others, though its effect may wear off after a few months. Some antidepressants like venlafaxine (Effexor) and desipramine (Norpramin) have stimulating properties, as does the antiseizure drug topiramate (Topamax). Stronger stimulants like methylphenidate (Ritalin, Concerta), and amphetamines (Dexedrine, Adderal) should probably only be used under the supervision of a psychiatrist.

Medications for Restless Legs Syndrome (RLS)

Given that RLS is unpleasant and interferes with quality sleep, it's important to treat it whenever it occurs. Probably the most commonly used medications for RLS are the anti-Parkinson's drugs pramipexole (Mirapex) and ropinirole (Requip). Other options include clonazepam (Klonopin), gabapentin (Neurontin), and levodopa/carbidopa (Sinemet).

Other Medications

Drugs can also play an important part in relieving symptoms other than pain and sleep problems. If you've been unfortunate enough to develop other symptoms such as irritable bowel syndrome or migraine headaches, you may need medications to combat those problems, too. For example, your doctor may prescribe tegaserod (Zelnorm) and alosetron (Lotronex) if you suffer from irritable bowel syndrome. If you have migraines, you may need a triptan. If you have interstitial cystitis, you may need to take pentosan polysulfate (Elmiron).

⌊, Essential

If you're tired of buying so many medications—only to find they don't work—ask your doctor for samples. Pharmaceutical sales reps provide samples to physicians regularly. You should also call your doctor for samples to tide you over if you're out and waiting for delivery of your next bottle or package.

The challenge with medications is always to balance out the effectiveness with the side effects. Sometimes, you need to discontinue the first remedy and find a new one. In other cases, you may need to adopt a different regimen altogether. For most people, finding the right mix of medications is a lengthy process that requires patience.

Using Drugs Safely and Wisely

It's not at all unusual for people who have fibromyalgia to wind up taking several medications at once to treat all the different symptoms. Consider the case of Bridget.

Every single day for the last four years, Bridget has taken 80 mg of methadone for the achy flu-like pain she gets; 10 mg of Valium for her shaking; 5 mg of Ritalin to help her stay alert; 100 mg of Trazadone to help her sleep; 325 mg of Percocet for severe pain; and Colase, an over-the counter stool softener that helps with constipation from IBS. She also uses marijuana, which she gets from a neurologist, to help with nausea and pain. "I don't get high on any of my medications, which is why I take them," she says. "I also try to cut down or go off the Ritalin or Valium just to keep its efficacy so I don't have to increase it." Before taking any drug, she does research on the Internet to better understand how it works and to learn of a drug's side effects. "I never forget that living in chronic pain is just as harmful as any drugs that remove that pain," Bridget says.

For people like Bridget, the safe use of her medications is vital. When you're already wracked with pain and fatigue, the last thing you need is a problem with a medication you're taking. That's why it's so important to take your drugs wisely. Here are some steps you can take to ensure safe drug use.

Reveal All

Providing good, reliable information is critical when it comes to getting prescription medications. So don't hold back when your doctor asks what medications you are taking. Include everything, even acetaminophen, birth control pills, and your daily multivitamin. Tell him about the occasional herbal supplement such as Echinacea, which you might take with a cold.

And if you have allergies or other medical conditions, share that information, too. Certain medications are not well tolerated by people who have preexisting conditions. The information you provide will help your doctor pinpoint the best treatment for your case.

Follow Doctor's Orders

It's tempting to take a little more of a drug that's giving you the relief you're desperately seeking. It might also be tempting to take less on days when you feel better. Because the symptoms of fibromyalgia can fluctuate drastically, you may in fact be able to reduce or increase your dosage according to the severity of your symptoms. But you should never alter your dosage without talking to your doctor first. Also, never share your medication with anyone else.

Watch for Side Effects

Many medications produce side effects. Some are tolerable and a minor, temporary nuisance, while others are downright dangerous, even life threatening. Other side effects go away after a week or two, once your body has adjusted to the drug.

The key is spotting those that are potentially life threatening and warrant your doctor's attention. Some of the more serious side effects include nausea and vomiting, rapid or irregular heartbeat, rash or hives, hallucinations, lack of coordination, ringing in the ears, blurred vision, changes in your menstrual cycle, and changes in your sex drive, or impotence. You should also call your doctor if you develop an infection, swelling, or fever.

Dangerous Mixes

When taken in combination with other food and drugs, some medications can cause a serious interaction, with serious repercussions. For instance, combining cimetidine (Tagamet) with sertraline (Zoloft) can affect your heart and lead to sudden death. Even certain foods can be unsafe if eaten with particular drugs. Drinking grapefruit juice with an antihistamine for instance, can cause heart problems.

That's why it's critical that you tell your doctor about *all* medicines that you are taking, including over-the-counter remedies, vitamins, and herbal supplements. You should also ask about food interactions. Even better, get all your medications from one pharmacy, where the pharmacist filling out the prescription can see what else you are taking. If you forget to ask your doctor, you should ask your pharmacist about any potential interactions.

Fact

Food affects the action of a drug in several ways. It can impair absorption of vitamins and minerals, stimulate or suppress the appetite, and alter the way your body uses nutrients. But the impact of any food and drug interactions depends on your age, size, and health, as well as the dosage of the drug, and when the food is eaten and the drug is taken. In some cases, you may simply have to change the timing of your food or drug in order to avoid a bad interaction.

Store Them Safely

Many people store medications in bathroom cabinets. But in reality, moisture and heat from showers and baths can cause some medications to deteriorate, which can lessen their strength and effectiveness.

In fact, any place where the temperature fluctuates is a bad storage place for medications. That means you should not keep drugs in the glove compartment of your car, on a nightstand that sits in sunlight, or on the windowsill of your kitchen. You should also steer clear of kitchen cabinets near the stove or dishwasher, where temperatures can fluctuate. Instead, look for storage areas that remain at room temperature, which means 59 to 86 degrees Fahrenheit. Better options include a kitchen cabinet, a bedroom closet, or a dresser drawer.

Of course, for some people, the bathroom might still be the most convenient place, especially if you take your medicines at night. In that case, make sure the containers are tightly sealed to prevent any moisture from seeping in. Wherever they wind up, make sure the drugs are placed on high shelves away from young children. Store all medications in their original containers, and throw out any that have expired.

Take Them Cautiously

When you do take a drug, be sure to let someone know what you are taking. That way, if you do have a bad reaction, someone will be on hand to let your doctor know in the event you can't. Be sure to measure the medication with the right spoon or cup—dinner spoons aren't a good idea—and to follow the instructions exactly. Always take a medication with plenty of water. And if the label tells you to take it with food or without food, be sure to follow those instructions.

Consult Your Pharmacist

The pharmacist who hands you your medication is more than someone in a white lab coat who measures out your drugs. He is also a valuable source of information. According to the Institute for Safe Medication Practices, you should know the answer to several questions before you leave your pharmacy:

- What are the brand and generic names of the medications?
- What does it look like?
- Why am I taking it?
- How much should I take, and how often?
- When is the best time to take it?
- How long will I need to take it?
- What side effects should I expect, and what should I do if they happen?
- What should I do if I miss a dose?
- Does this interact with my other medications or any foods?

- Does this replace anything else I was taking?
- Where and how do I store it?

Some pharmacists dispense lengthy details about the medication that answer these questions. If not, ask your pharmacist for more information.

 Alert

Whether it's from the Internet or a foreign trip, don't buy drugs from other countries. Some of these medications may be dangerous. They are generally not manufactured according to the strict approval standards of the FDA, and may even contain untested substances that are considered illegal in the United States.

A Word on Over-the-Counter (OTC) Drugs

Somehow, a prescription drug seems more dangerous than one that you can simply pick up in the aisle of your nearest drugstore or supermarket. But in reality, over-the-counter (OTC) remedies can also be dangerous. For instance, taking more than 4,000 mg of acetaminophen (Tylenol) a day—the equivalent of eight extra-strength tablets—can lead to liver damage, even death.

When you do buy over-the-counter medications, read the labels carefully. Some might contain ingredients you should not be taking. Certain ingredients might interact with your other medications or cause an allergic reaction. Others might not be appropriate for treating your symptoms. If you have any trouble selecting the right product, always ask the pharmacist for help.

Choosing the Right One(s)

Pinning down the medication regimen that works for you takes time and trial and error. Some drugs might produce added benefits that might make them superior to other therapies. Others might have side effects or interactions with other drugs that you don't want to tolerate. For instance, doxepin (Sinequan) is a tricyclic that has an antihistamine and can help people with allergies. But fluoxetine (Prozac) may not be a good choice if you have trouble sleeping, since it can be stimulating.

And remember, just when you think you've found the right combination, your symptoms might change. It is simply the nature of fibromyalgia. That's why it's so important to remain watchful for any side effects or changes in how well a medication works. In some cases, the medicine you take may become less effective over time because your body has become better at breaking it down. When that happens, your doctor may need to put you on a different drug.

CHAPTER 11

Alternative Fibro Treatments

A government survey in 2004 found that 36 percent of American adults now use some form of complementary and alternative medicine (CAM), with the number rising to 62 percent when prayer and megavitamin therapy are included. For people who have fibromyalgia, some of these techniques have been a godsend, a lifesaver in the ongoing battle against pain and fatigue. Read on and find out if one of these therapies might work for you.

What Is CAM?

CAM stands for complementary and alternative medicine. "Complementary" refers to therapies used alongside conventional therapies, and "alternative" means medical practices that come from outside mainstream Western medicine. You may also hear the term "integrative medicine," which refers to the practice of using therapies that treat mind and spirit as well as the body and which we'll explore in Chapter 16.

Many of these practices may seem new to Americans, but in reality they have been in use for thousands of years. Several factors have given rise to the growing popularity of CAM therapies. Many people turn to CAM because traditional treatments haven't produced satisfactory results. They may experiment with CAM out of curiosity or out of concern about the overuse of pharmaceutical medications. Some believe—sometimes mistakenly—that CAM therapies are safer and less likely to cause side effects. And a growing body of research is demonstrating the effectiveness of specific alternative therapies, giving credence to what some cultures have known for centuries, that some of these remedies can really work.

Fact

A survey by the National Center for Complementary and Alternative Medicine and the National Center for Health Statistics found that CAM is most popular among people suffering from chronic pain. The survey also found that women are more likely than men to use CAM therapies, which are generally more popular among people who are better educated, have been hospitalized in the past year, and are former smokers.

But not all therapies work for everyone. Most are used as complementary treatments, as adjuncts to traditional drug therapies, exercise, and lifestyle modifications. Some may provide only temporary relief. If you decide that you'd like to give complementary therapies a try, talk to your physician first and proceed with caution. Just because something is alternative and natural does not mean that it is definitely safe and effective.

Acupuncture

Traditional Chinese medicine teaches that the body has patterns of energy flow that are essential for good health. When that energy—which the Chinese call qi (pronounced chi)—is disrupted, a person's health falters. Acupuncture helps to restore that flow with the insertion of tiny needles along meridian lines on the body, which correspond to various organs. The procedure is believed to work by opening up the pathways of qi and restoring health.

Acupuncture originated in China more than 3,000 years ago. Here in the United States, it has become a popular method for alleviating all kinds of pain. As a treatment for fibromyalgia, study results have been mixed. But for those who have had success, acupuncture may work by inducing relaxation and promoting sleep, which in turn can benefit your pain. The procedure may be also used to relieve migraines, to enhance fertility, and to alleviate depression.

The Treatment

During an acupuncture session, a practitioner will insert as many as fifteen thin needles into specific points on your body. The location of each needle corresponds to the site of your pain, but it is not necessarily inserted in the place where you hurt. The needles do not draw blood and, in most cases, do not cause much pain. But you may feel a prick at insertion. Each acupuncture session lasts about an hour, and patients generally need four to six sessions before seeing results.

For people who do not like needles, acupressure offers an alternative. Acupressure involves the same principles as acupuncture. But instead of needles, the procedure involves the use of the practitioner's hands.

If you do decide to try acupuncture, find a licensed therapist, preferably one who has treated people with fibromyalgia before. Discuss your plans with your doctor to make sure you're healthy enough. Be honest with the acupuncturist about your health; he should be told of your fibromyalgia as well as other conditions and any medications you take. If your acupuncturist recommends herbal supplements, talk to your doctor first before taking them. They could cause dangerous interactions. Also, keep track of your progress. Acupuncture may require four to six sessions before it takes effect.

Acupuncture is not likely to cause side effects, but your practitioner is obligated by law to use sterile needles that have never been used before. Unsterilized needles can put you at risk for infection.

Trigger-Point Therapy

Fibromyalgia is characterized by the presence of tender points, but some people find relief with trigger-point therapy, also called myotherapy or myofascial therapy. As you might recall, trigger points are tight, highly irritable spots in a taut band of muscle that can cause referred pain, or pain located away from the trigger point itself.

Many people confuse trigger points and tender points. Trigger points are spastic knots in the muscles that cause pain. Tender points are the spots doctors press to determine if you have fibromyalgia. Virtually everyone has trigger points, though they may not be active.

Since fibro causes increases pain sensitivity, fibro patients are much more sensitive to their trigger points than normal people. The pain caused by the trigger point makes the person tighten her muscles, thereby creating more trigger points around her body in a "brush fire" effect. In many fibro patients, this can be a major part of the pain they're experiencing. That's why trigger-point therapy is helpful.

Trigger-point therapy uses a combination of stretching and deep manual pressure applied to specific trigger points to relax the knotted muscles and break the cycle of pain. It's often combined with heat, ice, cold spray, ultrasound, or electrical stimulation to make it more effective and to encourage the tissue to respond to the treatment.

Alert

In your quest for relief, you may be tempted to give magnets a try. Magnet manufacturers claim that magnets relieve pain and stimulate blood flow. But there is absolutely no evidence that any of these products work to relieve fibromyalgia. Your best bet: Save your money for a more proven therapy.

To treat the affected trigger points, the practitioner applies pressure using fingers, knuckles, and/or elbows to each point for up to thirty seconds. You may initially feel pain from the pressure, but it should never cross the line between "good" pain and "bad" pain. The therapy usually leads to considerable relief.

During treatment, it's very important to tell the therapist if the treatment starts to hurt. Pressure that's too aggressive can activate the trigger point, setting off a spasm and increasing the pain.

In severe cases, trigger-point injections can be added to the treatment. If done by themselves, the effect of injections tends to be more temporary. Though some doctors still put steroid medications in the shots, this generally is not recommended. Steroids provide minimal additional benefit and can cause side effects.

It's also very important to have your practitioner teach you how to treat yourself. Myofascial self-care, done twice a day, can dramatically increase your rate of improvement and gives you some control over your own pain. Eventually, you can become good enough at it that you won't need another person to do it for you.

Chiropractics

Until recent years, chiropractics was regarded with skepticism by traditional medicine. But like many alternative treatments, chiropractics has been around for centuries in one form or another. Here in the United States, chiropractics was popularized by Daniel David Palmer in the late 1800s. Palmer believed that the body had a powerful ability to heal itself, and that this ability was sustained by the proper flow of impulses coming from the nerves. Any misalignment of the spine, however, disrupted this flow. If an organ didn't receive the normal supply of impulses, it became diseased. Manipulating the spine therefore helped to correct the misalignment and bring about healing.

Today, chiropractics has become popular for the treatment of pain, especially lower back pain. But it can also improve headache pain, temporomandibular joint disorder, and chronic myofascial pain. Some people visit chiropractors for reasons besides musculoskeletal pain, such as preventing colds, alleviating allergies, and improving body mechanics.

Despite its growing acceptance, not everyone is convinced that chiropractics works. In fact, some say the evidence for its efficacy in the treatment of fibromyalgia is weak. Whether it will work for you will depend on how fibromyalgia is affecting you. Some people may find that while chiropractics does not alleviate pain, it can relieve fatigue and improve sleep.

Seeing a Chiropractor

Chiropractors are not medical doctors; rather, they receive a doctor of chiropractic degree upon graduating from an accredited school. On your first visit, you'll provide a patient history and undergo a physical exam. When the chiropractor does an actual treatment, he will do an adjustment using his hands. These adjustments involve applying a controlled sudden force to the joint, often the spine. Afterwards, you may notice some discomfort, but many people say they feel better after a visit to the chiropractor.

Alert

A chiropractic visit may not be the best treatment if you're suffering from neck pain. A technique known as cervical spinal manipulation, or neck cracking, has been linked to an increased risk for stroke. If you do suffer from neck pain, talk to your doctor about other treatments, such as analgesics or exercise.

To find a good chiropractor, ask around for a referral. There are about 50,000 licensed chiropractors in the United States. Make sure the chiropractor attended an accredited college and is licensed to practice in your state.

The effectiveness of chiropractors varies widely. Some can help fibro patients significantly, while others manhandle them and leave them much worse than before the treatment. Be sure that you find one who has helped other fibro patients.

Some people, like Alison, found relief with a chiropractor who did motion palpation.

The first chiropractor Alison saw never adjusted her at all and instead told her she was 85 percent disabled and that there was nothing he could do. Three years later, still in excruciating pain, Alison tried another chiropractor, who told her he'd never seen so many locked up joints in his life. The second chiropractor then went from joint to joint, and adjusted each one. For Alison, the right chiropractor greatly reduced her fibro pain and improved her mobility.

Not everyone, however, is a candidate for chiropractics. If you have a recent fracture, osteoporosis, rheumatoid arthritis, or neurological problems, you should avoid chiropractors. Also, chiropractors are not eligible to prescribe medications, but they may suggest other alternative therapies such as heat and ice, homeopathy, and dietary supplements.

Massage

For most people, a massage is a luxury. Many people can't afford the cost of a regular massage, and health insurance companies generally don't cover massages. But for some people, massage is therapy. Massage is the manual manipulation of soft body tissues. Rubbing, kneading, rolling, and pressing the tissue increases blood flow and warmth, relieves muscle tension, and promotes relaxation. Try giving yourself a massage, or have your partner do it for you. Gently massaging your own muscles can help relieve tension, especially in your face and head. But done too rigorously or for too long or short of a time, massage may cause pain. The key is to be gentle. If you're too aggressive, you can cause a flare.

In people who have fibromyalgia, massage can help alleviate pain, stiffness, and tight muscles. And by improving blood flow, the body can better deliver essential nutrients and oxygen to affected tissues, while flushing out toxins that might perpetuate your pain. Different types of massage can produce somewhat different results. The following sections describe just a few examples of the kinds you might consider.

Swedish Massage

A Swedish massage focuses on the soft tissues near the surface of your skin and doesn't involve heavy pressure needed to reach the soft tissue deeper in your body.

During a Swedish massage, the therapist uses a smooth, flowing style with long strokes and kneading movements that promotes relaxation, improves circulation, and relieves muscular tension. In fibro patients, a Swedish massage can be relaxing, but its benefits are generally short-lived.

Deep Tissue Massage

When muscles are tense and inflexible, some people may opt for a deep tissue massage. Deep tissue massages are more vigorous and are designed to loosen hardened or inflexible muscles and nearby tissues. The strokes are typically slow and methodic, and they may either go with or against the grain of the muscles.

Some say that deep tissue massage improves some symptoms of fibromyalgia, but only temporarily. In many people, deep tissue massage is too aggressive, leaving them sore and miserable.

Essential

Try heat and cold for achy muscles. Heat from a shower or bath can relax the muscles, decrease pain, and improve flexibility. Cold in the form of ice packs can ease pain if you suffer from nerve entrapment. But avoid heat and cold if you are sensitive to temperature extremes.

Myofascial Release

Myofascial release targets the fascia, or the soft thin tissue that covers every organ of our body. The technique is done to relieve tightness and restricted movement in the body's fibrous or connective tissue. This is especially beneficial for fibromyalgia sufferers since this disorder involves the fibrous tissue. The long stretching strokes of myofascial release can actually lengthen connective tissue and reduce its pull on the skeletal system, providing much-needed relief.

The Right Massage

The massage you choose will depend on several factors, including individual preference and pain tolerance. Whatever you decide, find a practitioner who knows about fibromyalgia and who is nationally certified by the National Certification Board for Therapeutic Massage and Bodywork, or one who has graduated from a training program certified by the Commission on Massage Therapy Accreditation.

On your first visit, let your massage therapist know you have fibromyalgia and work with her to find a pressure that is relaxing. If it hurts, let her know. Too much pressure causes muscles to tense. Although massage is almost always safe, do steer clear if you have inflammation, swelling, open sores, or circulation problems.

Reiki

Many alternative practitioners believe that everyone is endowed with a form of universal energy. Channeling that energy for the purpose of healing is the premise behind reiki (means "spiritually guided life energy"), an ancient Japanese healing art.

Reiki has been practiced for thousands of years throughout Japan, China, and other Asian nations. In recent years it has gained so much popularity in the United States that the National Center for Complementary and Alternative Medicine recently funded a study in Seattle to look at the impact of reiki on fibromyalgia.

According to the International Center for Reiki Training, reiki responds to the way we think and feel. When we consciously or unconsciously accept negative thoughts or feelings about ourselves, these thoughts attach themselves to our energy field and disrupt the flow of our life force, causing ill health.

Reiki heals by altering the energy field and charging it with positive energy. The healing is done with the help of a trained reiki master. As the negative energy breaks apart and falls away, the affected energy pathways are healed, and the life force can resume flowing in a healthy and natural way. Exactly how reiki works is unclear, but proponents tout it as an effective form of therapeutic touch, one that can promote relaxation, relieve pain, and reduce emotional distress.

Getting Reiki

During a reiki treatment, the client typically lies fully clothed on a massage table, though treatments can also be given in a sitting or standing position. The reiki practitioner places his hands on or near your body in different positions. His hands may be around your neck and shoulders, near your stomach, or on your feet. Other positions may be used as well, depending on your symptoms. Each position is held for three to ten minutes, and the whole treatment usually lasts between forty-five and ninety minutes.

Individual experiences with reiki vary, but almost everyone reports feeling more relaxed. Some people say they feel a glowing radiance around them, and a feeling of peace and well-being. Others may drift off to sleep or have an out-of-body experience.

If you are interested in reiki, discuss it with your physician first. Although reiki may not relieve you of all your fibro symptoms, it may provide you with the relaxation you need to help you sleep better and lessen your pain. For more information on reiki, check out the International Center for Reiki Training Web site at *www.reiki.org.*

Herbal Supplements

Nip a cold. Boost your energy. Relieve your anxiety. More and more, people are turning to herbal supplements in a quest for relief from anything that ails them, be it arthritis, depression, or the common cold, especially when traditional remedies fail them.

People who have fibromyalgia are likely candidates for taking herbal supplements. If you've been unable to achieve relief from pharmaceutical drugs or other therapies, you may wonder if these alternative remedies might do the trick.

The answer, unfortunately, is not clear. The science on many of these products is murky, and most people are left to rely on anecdotal reports about a supplement's effects. At the same time, some people do find success with herbal remedies. The key to taking any of these products is to approach with caution.

Safety First

Before we mention some of the more common products associated with the treatment of fibromyalgia, it's important to discuss the safety factor. Let's face it: People who have a chronic pain condition are vulnerable targets for unscrupulous marketers peddling cure-alls and therapies that promise relief.

Truth is, there is little scientific proof to back up many of these claims. Each treatment needs to be considered on its own merits and how it might impact your health. But you should keep some general guidelines in mind:

- "Natural" does not mean "safe." Think of the poisonous mushrooms and berries that grow in the wild.
- Everyone responds differently. The state of your health, how the treatment is used, even your belief in the treatment can all impact how well a remedy works for you.
- Beware of any health claims. Claims that a supplement can diagnose, treat, cure, or prevent disease are invalid and must have scientific proof. Without scientific evidence, such claims violate regulations, and the product is considered an unapproved drug.
- Stick with established manufacturers. They can be held accountable for their products.
- If you use herbal products, be sure they're "standardized." This means that they've been measured and guarantee the amount of active ingredient in the pill, not just the amount of the herb.

Keep in mind too that supplements are classified as food, not drugs. The U.S. Food and Drug Administration regulates dietary supplements under the Dietary Supplement Health and Education Act of 1994 (DSHEA), which says the dietary supplement manufacturer is responsible for ensuring that a supplement is safe before it is marketed. Safety depends on several factors, including the ingredients, where they come from, and the quality of the manufacturing process. Manufacturers must also make sure that information on the label is truthful and not misleading.

Most manufacturers do not need to register with the FDA or get FDA approval before producing or selling dietary supplements. The FDA is responsible, however, for taking action against any unsafe dietary supplement product after it reaches the market. So if a product is deemed unsafe, the FDA can prohibit its sale.

Essential

When buying supplements, look for products with the USP seal. The U.S. Pharmacopeia is the standards-setting authority for all prescription and over-the-counter drugs and supplements. With supplements, the USP ensures what's on the label is in the bottle, in the proper amounts and without contaminants. It also makes sure the supplement will release the active ingredients into the body and that the manufacturing practices are safe.

Popular Supplements for Fibro

It's not unusual at all for fibro sufferers to turn to supplements. While it would be impossible to list every supplement that you might consider taking, you should be familiar with some that seem to have some benefit to people with fibromyalgia. Keep in mind, though, that not all supplements will help all patients. Again, it will take some trial and error to pin down those that work for you.

Coenzyme Q10

Popularly known as CoQ10, coenzyme Q10 is naturally produced in the body. It is used in the production of cellular energy and as a disease-combating antioxidant. In people with fibromyalgia, it might help relieve fibro fog.

DHEA

As a supplement, DHEA is a synthesized version of a hormone made by the adrenal glands that is a basic building block of many hormones. Often billed as an anti-aging remedy, DHEA is said to improve pain, fatigue, and depression. But a study in 2005 found that despite its popularity among fibro sufferers, DHEA showed no real benefit. It can also cause significant side effects.

Magnesium and Malic Acid

Magnesium is an essential mineral, and malic acid is a fruit acid found in apples. Together, they can stimulate the body's production of adenosine triphosphate, an energy source in many body cells that may be deficient in people with fibromyalgia.

Melatonin

Melatonin is a hormone secreted by the body that is involved in regulating our sleep-wake cycles. Some people believe that FMS sufferers do not produce enough melatonin on their own at night. As a supplement, melatonin can sometimes induce sleep.

SAM-e

SAM-e, or adenosylmethionine, is a natural substance that may relieve pain and depression. In the body, it helps produce and regulate hormones that affect mood. Research on SAM-e in fibro patients has been mixed, but some believe it relieves pain, fatigue, and depression. SAM-e is very expensive, and any benefit requires very high doses.

St. John's Wort

This popular remedy is hailed as a treatment for depression. Although commonly used in Europe, experts in the United States say it is effective in treating only mild depression. It should never be taken with other antidepressants, and it may interact with other medications as well.

Chlorella

Studies show that Chlorella pyrenoidosa, a freshwater algae that evolved more than 2 billion years ago, may relieve the symptoms of fibromyalgia.

Ginseng

Panax ginseng has been used for thousands of years in Asia to treat fatigue. Many fibro sufferers find it helps with mental energy and motivation. But it can be overstimulating and cause high blood pressure as well as sleep problems.

5-HTP

5-HTP is one chemical step away from serotonin, a major neurotransmitter. Many find that taking it at bedtime helps sleep, and higher doses may also help depression. But it should never be taken if you're on antidepressants.

Peppermint Oil

Enteric-coated peppermint oil—which means the active ingredient is not released until the pill is past your stomach—has been found by many people to help irritable bowel syndrome.

Feverfew

Feverfew is an herb that may reduce the frequency and severity of migraines, but responses vary widely.

Other Possibilities

You may encounter other supplements for the treatment of fibro symptoms such as valerian for anxiety, gingko biloba for memory and brain function, vitamin C for immune function, milk thistle for liver cleansing, and alpha lipoic acid for detoxification.

Doing the Research

Before taking any supplement or engaging in any alternative therapy, learn the potential risks and benefits, and discuss your plans with your health-care practitioners. Tell them about the therapy you are considering and ask about its safety, effectiveness, and interactions with medications you're taking. Even if your doctor can't give you specifics, he might be able to refer you to someone who can. You can also ask your doctor to interpret the information you do find. A good place to start is the Internet. The Web may be the source of some outlandish health claims, but it's also a wonderful resource for information. Some good places to check include the following:

- The National Center for Complementary and Alternative Medicine Web site, at *www.nccam.nih.gov*. Information is provided about specific therapies, and you can find out whether there are new or ongoing studies into the treatment.
- The FDA, at *www.fda.gov*. If you're looking into dietary supplements, check out the FDA's Center for Food Safety and Applied Nutrition Web site at *www.cfsan.fda.gov*. Or visit the FDA's Web page on recalls and safety alerts at *www.fda.gov*.
- The Federal Trade Commission (FTC), at *www.ftc.gov*. Examine fraudulent claims or consumer alerts regarding various therapies.
- The Diet, Health, and Fitness Consumer Information Web site, at *www.ftc.gov/bcp/menu-health.htm*.
- Complementary and Alternative Medicine on PubMed, at *www.nlm.nih.gov/nccam/camonpubmed.html*. Citations or abstracts (brief summaries) are provided for study results on alternative therapies.
- The International Bibliographic Information on Dietary Supplements, at *www.ods.od.nih.gov*. Search the scientific literature on dietary supplements.
- ConsumerLab.com. Information is provided to evaluate health products, such as supplements.

When you're evaluating information you get from the Web, check to see that the operator of the site is the government, a university, or a reputable medical or health-related association. Be wary if the site belongs to a company that manufactures or sells the supplement. Also be sure the information is current and based on scientific evidence. The material should present clear references to back it up, not opinions.

To help you weed out good supplements from the bad ones, you may want to enlist the help of an integrative medicine physician. A good Web site for help in locating a doctor is *www.holisticmedicine.org*.

Diet Know-How

It would be great if there were a specific dietary regimen that could wipe out your symptoms of fibromyalgia. Truth is, there is no single diet plan, food, or nutrient that will relieve your pain and fatigue. Anyone who claims that there is a dietary cure is misleading you. But that doesn't mean that eating well won't help. In fact, it's always advisable to eat a well-balanced diet, rich in nutrients and limited in unhealthy fats and sugars. A good diet helps reduce your risk for disease, strengthens your immune system, and ensures that your body performs at its best.

Essential Nutrients

People with fibromyalgia should take steps to ensure they get certain nutrients. Some of these nutrients can help relieve their symptoms. Certain vitamins and minerals warrant special attention:

- B vitamins assist in energy metabolism, brain functions and neurological health. These are found in fortified foods, leafy greens, eggs, fish, milk, and other foods.
- Vitamin A is an antioxidant that can improve vision. It can be found in orange-colored fruits and vegetables such as sweet potatoes, carrots, and apricots.
- Vitamin C is another antioxidant that enhances immunity. It can be found in citrus fruits and numerous vegetables.

- Magnesium is a mineral that assists in muscle contractions and energy production. It can be found in nuts, legumes, and whole grains.
- Calcium is a mineral involved in bone formation and proper muscle function. It can be found in dairy products, leafy greens, and fortified foods.
- Potassium is a mineral that aids in nerve transmission and muscle function. It can be found in fruits, vegetables, and chicken.

A Healthy Diet

Eating healthy is always important, but when you're sick, a good diet is critical. Fill your plate with nutrient-dense foods such as vegetables, fruits, and complex carbohydrates. These foods contain important antioxidants and other disease-fighting substances. When choosing meat, stick with leaner varieties such as chicken, fish, and turkey. Make sure to get a balance of carbohydrates and protein. Your body needs both nutrients to stay well.

At the same time, reduce your intake of saturated fat and cholesterol, which can promote heart disease and weight gain. Avoid processed foods. These are often made with refined sugar and partially hydrogenated oils that contain trans-fatty acids, which have been linked to heart disease. Drink alcohol in moderation, or not at all if you're taking medications. Many experts also recommend steering clear of sugar, artificial sweeteners, preservatives, additives, and caffeine—all substances that can aggravate your fibro symptoms.

Some people with fibromyalgia notice they are sensitive to specific foods. To figure out the offending food, do an elimination diet, which involves eating a specific diet, and then gradually reintroducing suspect foods to figure out which ones trigger your symptoms. For specifics, check out the elimination diet offered by the CFIDS Association of America at *www.cfids.org*. Many people who have irritable bowel syndrome find that they do better if they eliminate glutens, a protein found in wheat and other grains. You can find many gluten-free diets on the Internet. If you are plagued by severe intestinal symptoms, consider trying one of these diets for a week or two. For those who'd rather not abide by a diet, try eliminating the most common allergy triggers, such as milk, wheat, eggs, citrus, and chocolate. To learn more about diet, consult a nutritionist.

CHAPTER 12

Living with Fibromyalgia

The myriad ways that fibro impacts day-to-day life varies markedly from one patient to the next. One person might find it impossible to do her job. Another might still be able to garden with no problem. Still another might have trouble preparing meals. The effects of fibromyalgia on your daily life also change as your symptoms do. But you can take steps to minimize the impact of your condition.

Adapting to Fibromyalgia

Learning to live with fibromyalgia requires that you first adapt to the idea that you have a chronic illness. That means you will have to accept this new condition and the fact that you may not be able to return to your previous state of health. For some, the situation can be devastating.

According to Patricia Fennell, MSW, author of *The Chronic Illness Workbook: Strategies and Solutions for Taking Back Your Life,* adapting to chronic illness is a four-phase process that involves crisis, stabilization, resolution, and integration. Here is a summary of the phases, based on an article by Fennell that appeared on the National Fibromyalgia Association Web site.

Crisis

In the early stage of illness, you are seized by overwhelming emotions that leave you fretful about what is happening. Could you be dying? Are you mentally ill? What will become of your family? As your symptoms gradually worsen or interfere with your daily life, you become increasingly frustrated. If diagnosis doesn't come quickly, you may start to feel more isolated and worried, concerned that you're losing your mind. Friends and family may regard you with worry, suspicion, disbelief, or loving support, all of which may affect the way you endure this early stage.

Stabilization

Gradually, you start to become accustomed to the illness. By now, you may even have a diagnosis, which gives you something to work with. But you may be having a hard time adapting to the notion that you are not well, so you may try to become normal again. When it doesn't happen, you may become frustrated.

Essential

Knowing as much as you can about fibromyalgia—or any condition—can actually improve your health. According to the National Institute of Arthritis and Musculoskeletal and Skin Diseases, studies have shown that rheumatoid arthritis (RA) patients who are well informed and actively participate in their care have less pain and make fewer visits to the doctor than others with RA. Although the research looked at RA, the same applies to other medical conditions.

The people around you are also coming to terms with your physical limitations. Some may be supportive, but others may be cold, even callous, and say things that are hurtful. As a result, you may withdraw. You may even slip backwards into the crisis phase. Around this time, too, you may be launching the process of educating yourself about fibromyalgia. You might even seek out a support group, or a better doctor. In the back of your mind, you are hopeful of resuming some semblance of normalcy. When that does not happen, you enter the next stage.

Resolution

Unable to resume normalcy, you begin to accept your new self. You may start to question what has happened to you at this point. Why am I sick? What can I do now? What is left for me to do?

During this stage, which can often be quite difficult emotionally, many people realize they need extra support, possibly from close friends, but also from a trusted clergy person or a professional counselor. These people can help you find meaning in what has happened and put you on a new path that incorporates your new identity. As you emerge from this phase, you realize that you do have hopes for a new future, perhaps different from the one you imagined.

By now, you realize that there is no cure and begin to accept that the best route is to build a new identity. On the way, you may renew some friendships, but you may also lose others. You may find yourself making new friends, cutting back on your job responsibilities, and taking on new creative projects, such as writing or drawing, that help you find meaning in this new life.

Integration

The passage of time has taught you valuable lessons about fibromyalgia and its cyclical, evolving nature. When you suffer a flare-up, you're now better equipped to deal with it, even to accept it as part of your new life. So while your body may still be wracked with pain, you are better able mentally to cope.

Question

How do I support a friend with fibromyalgia?
A friend's support can make a world of difference to how someone with fibromyalgia feels. Be patient and considerate, and offer to help with chores and errands. Spend time with your friend doing activities she can do comfortably. Offer to accompany her to doctor's appointments. But beware of telling her how good she looks, because she probably feels lousy.

By this point, your illness is not the only thing that defines you. You have fully integrated your condition into your existence. You also have new friends—and possibly resumed relations with old friends—

who know you as someone with fibromyalgia, but who do not define you solely by your condition.

The Phase You're In

Now that you know the four phases, ask yourself these questions. Where are you in the process of adapting to fibromyalgia? What can you do to get to the final stage of integration? Whether you're trapped in the first phase of crisis or working on the third phase of resolution, it's important to recognize that you can live, and even live well, with chronic illnesses like fibromyalgia. There are things you can do each and every day that will help you do that.

Listening to Your Body

Before you had fibromyalgia, you were probably able to get away with pushing yourself beyond your capabilities. If you were up against a deadline, you could stay up until midnight for a week and get the job done. But now that you have fibromyalgia, staying up late and multi-tasking may feel like daunting challenges.

It's critical that you heed what your body is telling you, which is "Stop—I need my rest." That means you may need to find new ways of doing things, strategies that will conserve your energy and minimize your pain.

One of the difficulties with fibro is that you often won't know you've overdone it until the next day. When this happens, look back on your previous day's activities, and try to get a sense of how you overdid it. Then, avoid doing too much in the future, even though you may not feel tired at the time.

Body Mechanics

Few of us pay much attention to the way we walk, sit, or stand when we perform these simple everyday activities. We simply do it. But proper body mechanics—which means keeping your skeleton in good alignment—are important, especially when your body is in pain. The key is to move and perform in ways that do not aggravate pain.

Sitting at Work

These days, many people spend hours sitting at a computer or desk. Even if you don't work at a desk, you might have one at home where you work on a computer for research, entertainment, or e-mailing friends. But if you practice poor body mechanics at your desk or don't have an ergonomically sound setup, you could be causing your body added stress, strain, and pain.

In order to minimize pain caused from your workstation, it's important to make sure your chair and desk are properly adjusted and that you use them correctly. For starters, make sure your desk is elbow high. Adjust your computer screen so that it is eighteen to thirty inches from your eyes, or at about arm's length, and directly centered in front of you. Position your keyboard so that your forearms are parallel to your thighs when your feet are flat on the floor. And if you use the phone a lot, get one that has a headset. Other tips for desk workers include these:

- Keep objects you use regularly within easy reach.
- When sitting, make sure your knees are level with your hips.
- Use a swivel chair so that you can turn to talk to someone and not twist your body.
- Keep wrists straight and neutral when typing, and don't let them bend up, down, or to the side.
- Consider using voice recognition software to reduce your typing needs.
- Use your entire arm, not just your hand, when you move a mouse.
- Take short breaks and stretch your arms and fingers.

Driving

Make sure to position your seat so that you are close enough to the steering wheel without stretching and are still safe. Sit with your knees level with your hips. To support your lower back, use a rolled-up towel or commercial back support.

Kitchen Duty

Standing for long periods at a time at a kitchen counter can become a strain on anyone with aches and pains. Try propping one foot on a small footstool, an open drawer, or the ledge of an open cabinet door while you're standing. Make sure to stand up straight (see below). Use food processors, mixers, and other tools to reduce the wear and tear on your arms. Do some tasks sitting, if possible. Prepare foods ahead of time whenever you can. This will break up kitchen chores into smaller jobs that require less time.

Power of Posture

Turns out that Mom was right when she admonished you to stand up straight. Good posture is critical to proper body mechanics and the prevention of unnecessary strain on your muscles, joints, and ligaments. Whether you're sitting at your desk, driving your car, or walking to your mailbox, good posture puts your body in the least stressful position and makes it most efficient. Good posture also frees your muscles from holding your body in positions that can cause strain and pain. In addition, it helps you breathe better and distributes your weight more evenly.

 Alert

Poor posture does more than make you look bad. As you age, it can also cause numerous health problems, including decreased lung capacity, lower back pain, poor bowel function, and temporomandibular joint disorder. If that doesn't convince you to straighten up, consider this: Bad posture also makes you look older.

To improve your posture, begin by relaxing your entire body. Be on the lookout for muscle tension in the chin, the neck, and the shoulders, all areas that are likely to tense up. If you catch a muscle tightening up, take a deep breath and remind yourself to relax. To figure out whether you have good posture, look at yourself in the mirror while sitting or standing. Experiment with how you hold your body and the ways you move. Pay attention to any discomfort in your muscles as you bend, twist, and sit or stand. Sometimes, simply staying in one position for too long can cause pain.

Standing

Picture a straight line that connects your ears, shoulders, hips, knees, and heels. Keep your head over your shoulders, your shoulders over your pelvis, and your knees relaxed and unlocked. Tighten your tummy without overdoing it, and tuck in your buttocks. Place feet slightly apart, with one foot a little in front of the other for balance. Switch feet every twenty minutes or so, or change to a sitting position.

If you need to stand on a hard surface, wear shoes with good support and cushioning. If you still experience discomfort, sit down.

Sitting

The key to a proper sitting position is support for the spine. To do that, use pillows or a rolled-up towel to support your lower back. Keep shoulders back and chin tucked in a comfortable position. Your hips, knees, and ankles should all be at ninety-degree angles.

Sleeping

Sleeping in bad positions can cause unpleasant stress, strain, and pain in different parts of the body. A bad mattress can also cause pain. Different people like different types. Some people prefer waterbeds. Others like sheep's-wool mattress pads or body-conforming foam pads. Try several different types to see what works best for you. It's usually best to sleep on a mattress that is neither too hard nor too soft. You can take steps to minimize pain no matter how you sleep.

Back Sleepers

People who sleep on their back should place a cervical pillow or a small rolled-up towel under their neck to prevent neck strain. A pillow under the knees can help prevent lower back pain.

Side Sleepers

Place several soft pillows or a large body pillow under your arms and legs for added support. Be sure your pillow keeps your neck straight.

Stomach Sleepers

It's best to avoid sleeping on your stomach if you have fibromyalgia. This position reverses the natural curvature in your spine and can cause chronic muscle pain. If you absolutely cannot change your habit, place a pillow under your head to minimize neck rotation. Put another pillow under your stomach to prevent arching in your back.

Proper Muscle Use

The improper use of a muscle can set off your pain, too. That's why you should take steps to make sure you use your muscles correctly. Avoid lifting anything that is too heavy. When you do lift, hold the object close to your body, which will make the task less stressful. If you can, slide objects across the floor, so you don't have to lift them at all.

Essential

Lighten up—when you pack a purse. A heavy handbag can strain your neck and shoulder muscles. So stop toting around that mini-umbrella you never use, the unnecessary keys, and the excess makeup. Get in the habit of cleaning out your purse regularly so small items don't add up.

Whenever possible, use large muscles instead of small ones, like your palms instead of your fingers, and your arms instead of your hands. On the stairs, step up with your stronger leg. And always lift with stomach and large leg muscles, not your lower back. If you're carrying something heavy, switch arms frequently. The goal is to preserve the weaker, more vulnerable muscles. If you do have to carry fairly heavy loads frequently, consider using a wheeled airplane carry-on bag. When you do feel stiff or uncomfortable, shift positions. Get up, move around, and stretch your muscles, if possible. Remember, staying in one position for too long can also cause stiffness and pain.

Smart Pacing

When you're healthy, life is just one giant juggling act, filled with family and job responsibilities, volunteer duties, and social activities. In fact, that may be the way you like it, thank you very much.

But when you have a chronic illness like fibromyalgia, learning to pace yourself becomes important. For people accustomed to operating at a frenetic pace, slowing down can involve a major adjustment. It might take time and practice to accept that you can no longer do all that you want to do. But certain strategies can help.

Set Priorities

As irresistible as a new challenge may seem, you have to make your health your top priority. When you have fibromyalgia, you have to learn to say no and to do only those things that matter most. You also need to know when to ask for help. Of course, that doesn't mean you have to turn down every offer that comes your way or delegate absolutely everything. But it does mean being more picky about the tasks you do select. Treat your time and energy like money in a bank account—you only have so much, so you have to be careful how you spend it. Here are some good questions to ask yourself:

- Is this something I really want to do?
- Is this something I can realistically accomplish?
- Will taking on this project cause undue stress that could worsen my pain?
- Is there something else I can sacrifice if I do this?
- How much time will this involve?

Let the answers be your guide. You may find that taking on the project is not as good an idea as you thought and that it could compromise your health.

Plan Realistically

Most people keep calendars and to-do lists of what's coming up in the days or weeks ahead. For people who have fibromyalgia, plans can help you figure out what you must get done and what can wait. But when you're in the throes of severe pain, it might be hard to plan anything at all. You may not know how you'll feel two weeks from now, when your children want to visit an amusement park, or how you'll feel tomorrow when you're scheduled to give a presentation. Some days, planning to do nothing is a plan unto itself. Here are some tips on how to plan:

- Don't overdo it with a lengthy to-do list or a calendar jammed with activities.
- Always include time for rest and relaxation in your schedule.
- Alternate strenuous activities with less rigorous ones.
- Break up big jobs into smaller tasks.
- Do things in advance if you can.
- Try to always incorporate one pleasurable activity into your day.
- Avoid overplanning. It's impossible to predict how you'll feel a week from now, so focus getting through today.

Doing two or more things at once—or multitasking—may lead you to think you're accomplishing more. But studies show that people who multitask are actually losing time when they have to switch from one task to another, especially when the tasks are unfamiliar. Even worse, your ability to do either task is reduced when you try to do two at once. So get in the habit of doing one thing at a time.

Let's Get Practical

When you have fibromyalgia, concerns like a perfectly clean house may fall by the wayside, much to your horror and despair. The reality is that conserving your energy and minimizing your pain becomes much more important than how you look, how clean your house is, and whether you're preparing elaborate meals. With fibromyalgia, you need to become more practical. That might mean readjusting your values, making changes in your routine, and breaking some old habits.

Household Chores

For some people, doing routine household chores can become quite daunting in the face of fibromyalgia. And if you're accustomed to having a clean house, you may need to readjust your standards in order to cope with the rigors of managing your house.

Of course, the best answer to housework might be hiring outside help. But not everyone has the financial wherewithal to afford such a luxury. In the absence of outside help, you will need to adjust your housecleaning and standards to meet your health needs.

Break It Up

Do one heavy task each day instead of two or three in one day. Even better, break up a big task into several small ones, and spread them out over a few days. Rest frequently during longer or more strenuous tasks.

Minimize Clutter

Put everything back the instant you're done with it, and encourage family members to do the same. Toss out anything you no longer need or use. Eliminate junk mail by putting it in the recycling bin immediately.

Delegate

Even young children can help with household chores, like emptying wastepaper baskets or neatening hallways. Enlist your spouse or a friend to help with bigger chores.

Take Fewer Trips

Keep a basket near the stairs, and take up as much as you can easily carry at once instead of making several small trips.

Dress for Less Duress

On some days, the mere thought of getting dressed might be too painful to bear, much less the idea of washing, ironing, and hanging your clothes. When it comes to clothes, simplicity is the key. Avoid wearing clothes and shoes that are uncomfortable or too tight. Instead, choose loose, well-made clothes that are comfortable. To minimize clothing maintenance, do not buy garments that require hand washing, ironing, or dry cleaning.

Food Management

Preparing a meal might seem like a Herculean task to someone in the midst of a fibro flare. As much as you might enjoy eating a home-cooked meal, there will be days when you'll have to accept simpler dining, unless someone else can prepare it for you.

To help you get through the tough times, prepare meals and ingredients ahead of time—when you're feeling well—and store them in your freezer. In addition, consider using a slow cooker, which can save on the number of dishes you need to clean up.

Fact

For the person too tired to cook, canned foods are a healthy option. According to the American Dietetic Association, there are now more than 1,000 food items that come in a can. Best of all, canned foods are just as nutritious as their fresh and frozen counterparts.

You may need to rethink the way you shop for groceries, too. For instance, if you drive to several stores to take advantage of sales, you should consider the amount of time and energy you're expending simply to save a few dollars. In addition, you may need to purchase smaller items, which are not as heavy or bulky to carry.

On the worst days, consider ordering take-out or preparing canned or frozen foods, if you don't have someone to cook for you. Keep these kinds of foods handy in the event you have a bad day. As important as nutrition, such meals are occasionally necessary to help you get through a tough day.

A Safe House

No one wants to suffer a fall, and for a person with fibromyalgia, a bad fall could be a trigger that sets off a flare. That's why keeping your house safe and free of hazards is also important to your day-to-day existence. Here are a few tips:

- Eliminate scatter rugs.
- Provide enough light.
- Maintain steps and stairs.
- Remove clutter.
- Wear safe shoes (with nonskid soles and low heels).

Falls are the third leading cause of unintentional death in the Unites States, behind motor vehicle crashes and poisonings. In 2002, 14,500 people died in falls, according to the National Safety Council. More than 50 percent of all falls occur in the home. Most deaths caused by falls are associated with steps and stairs. The bottom line is to make sure your home is safe.

Assistive Devices

Some people may need assistive devices to make their homes and lives more fibro-friendly. Assistive devices are just what the name implies—products that can help you do tasks more easily. They're also helpful for people who have arthritis or other conditions that restrict mobility.

The types of assistive devices you need will depend on the level of your pain or disability. Talk to an occupational or physical therapist about where to find assistive devices. Consider putting them on your holiday wish list.

Attitude Counts

Okay, so you know when you hurt. You've even figured out the situations that worsen your pain. And you've taken steps to dress comfortably, limit your activity, and maintain a safe house. But you're still feeling a lot of pain—and a lot of anger about it.

When it comes to enduring the day-to-day rigors of fibromyalgia—or any chronic illness, for that matter—a positive attitude goes a long way. You might be wondering how you're supposed to stay positive when even dialing a phone hurts. Here are some tips that might help:

- Anticipate setbacks and the recovery that follows.
- Make a list of activities that truly distract you from the pain—and do them!
- Reach out to friends who are supportive.
- Count your blessings, and write them in a journal.
- Indulge yourself in something you usually don't.
- Consider the progress you've made and the lessons you've learned.

No doubt, staying positive is tough when you feel so bad. But a good attitude can help you persevere when the pain and fatigue of fibromyalgia becomes overwhelming.

CHAPTER 13

Staying Active

Exercise is probably the last thing you want to do when you're hurting. In reality, not exercising is one of the worst things you can do. Regular physical activity has myriad benefits for fibro sufferers. That doesn't mean you have to run or walk long distances, break a big sweat, or work out for long periods of time. In this chapter, we'll take a look at the best kinds of exercise for fibro sufferers and how physical activity can help you.

Why Exercise Matters

When you're suffering the pain and fatigue of fibromyalgia, exercise is probably as appealing as dinner with a bad boss. You might find it too difficult to even perform simple tasks like getting out of bed, climbing the stairs, or cooking a meal. Or you may find exercise too boring, inconvenient, and time consuming. Maybe you have simply never been in the habit of being active.

But for someone with fibromyalgia, exercise is a potent remedy for the pain and fatigue. Studies show that regular exercise, done safely, can work wonders to relieve pain, improve function, and enhance health. And experts agree that exercising two to four times a week can help fibro sufferers enjoy a better quality of life. Consider the perks that exercise provides:

- Makes you less stiff
- Improves sleep
- Strengthens muscles and decreases tension

- Makes it easier to do daily activities
- Relieves stress and anxiety
- Reduces depression
- Helps with weight control

On top of that, exercise enhances immunity, lowers blood pressure and cholesterol, and triggers the release of endorphins, which are your body's natural painkillers. Perhaps most important, exercise boosts your self-confidence and helps you gain a sense of control over your health.

Life Without Exercise

Avoiding physical activity can be the start of a vicious cycle, one that will only worsen your symptoms. The less you move, the weaker and smaller your muscles become. In addition, lack of activity will make your joints stiffer and increasingly inflexible, making it even harder for you to get the physical activity you need.

The lack of exercise can also worsen your depression, which is common among patients suffering from chronic pain. Feeling depressed can in turn make it harder to exercise. Next thing you know, you're trapped in a vicious cycle of pain, depression, and a lack of exercise, all of which will cause poor sleep, weight gain, and put you at risk for other health problems such as heart disease, diabetes, and even certain kinds of cancer (including breast, colon, and pancreas).

A similar cycle occurs with sleep as well. You don't sleep well, so you're too tired to exercise. But the less active you are, the worse your sleep becomes. That's why it's critical to do some physical activity, no matter how little you do or how insignificant it may seem. Gentle stretching, yoga, and short walks around the block can make an enormous difference to a body that's been wracked with pain. Talk to your doctor first before beginning any exercise program. You might even want to work with a physical therapist or a personal trainer familiar with fibromyalgia, either of whom can provide specific exercises that suit your condition.

Getting Started

Once you're inspired to start exercising, discuss your plans with your doctor. Ask him for recommendations on what you should do and whether he can recommend any health professionals to help you devise an enjoyable workout. When you do get out there, make sure to dress comfortably in loose-fitting clothes that don't restrict your movement in any way. Wear supportive shoes that absorb shock and do not allow slippage.

Alert

Choose a personal trainer who knows something about fibromyalgia. You should also find out whether a trainer is certified by a reputable national organization, such as the American Council on Exercise or the American College of Sports Medicine, and whether she's worked with other people with fibro. Consider asking for references, too. A good trainer won't mind having clients discuss her experience and skills.

The most common mistake fibromyalgia patients make is being too aggressive at first. This will cause a flare, leading you to mistakenly assume that exercise makes fibro worse. The key is to start low and proceed slow. Begin at about half of what you think you can do. If you don't notice a worsening of your fibro afterward, gradually build up your time by one to two minutes a day. When you reach a level that seems to cause your symptoms to worsen slightly the next day, back off a bit. Stay at the slower pace for a week or so, then start increasing again, but more slowly.

Try to exercise hard enough that you're breathing somewhat heavier but still able to carry on a conversation. If you can work out for up to twenty minutes a day, you'll reap most of the benefits that exercise offers fibro sufferers.

Begin any workout with a warm-up that involves gentle stretching. Never overdo any exercise, especially in the beginning when you are most vulnerable to injury. If you feel any discomfort at all, such as dizziness, severe shortness of breath, or tightness in your chest, stop immediately. You might want to try massaging any cramps. Resume exercising only if you think you can.

Finish any workout with a cool-down period. For instance, if you've been riding a stationary bike at a medium speed, bring it down to a slow one. Then do some gentle stretching without causing tension.

Types of Exercise

Often, when you think of exercise, you think of jogging, biking, or weight lifting. But physical fitness doesn't have to be that rigorous or so challenging. Exercise can also be gentle, slow, and rhythmic. To figure out the workout that's best for you, you should know the three basic types of exercise, all of which can play a role in improving your symptoms.

Range-of-Motion Exercises

Your range of motion is the range your joints can move in certain directions without causing pain. Any exercise that involves stretching and improving your flexibility fits in this category.

Essential

Getting a good stretch doesn't require an exercise mat or a large floor space. You can stretch at your desk, at a stoplight, or while you're preparing dinner. Shoulder circles, gentle arm reaches, and head turns can be done virtually anywhere, anytime. So if you're up for it, stop and stretch. Your body will thank you for it later.

Range-of-motion exercises are important to people who suffer from fibromyalgia. Regular stretching sustains joint mobility, reduces stiffness, and can make it easier for you to do everyday activities. It also elongates the ligaments and muscles around the joint, which will make these muscles more flexible. But a good stretch is also critical to the start of any activity you do. More than ever, your muscles need to be warmed up before a workout. Be sure, however, not to take it past the point of discomfort, which can cause a flare of pain in those muscles.

Since every patient is so different, you may have to try different workouts and activities before finding one that works for you. It's best however, to try and stretch every day. Good stretching exercises include yoga, tai chi, and qi gong, which all involve gentle stretching and deep breathing and give a meditative aspect to your workout.

Yoga

Yoga is an ancient practice that began in India 5,000 years ago. Although yoga can be a complete way of life, most people who practice yoga are engaged in doing asanas, or postures, which is known as hatha yoga. Hatha yoga also involves meditation and deep breathing. The movements are designed to improve flexibility, strengthen muscles, relax nerves, and promote circulation. The meditation and deep breathing can also reduce stress and anxiety, alleviate depression, and encourage better sleep.

For some people, like Danielle, yoga harnessed the mental awareness she needed to better understand her body's needs.

> Danielle was never good about listening to her body. She often did more than she should have and wound up in excruciating pain. At a friend's suggestion, she decided to give yoga a try. The slow movements accompanied by the gentle breathing made her more aware of what her body was feeling and taught her how to listen when it was urging her to take it easy. Now she knows when she can get away with doing more and when she needs to slow down.

The best time to practice yoga is at least two hours after a meal. Many people do it in the morning when they awaken or at night, before bed. If you awaken with morning stiffness, try taking a warm bath before doing your practice. Be careful, however. Many yoga instructors teach a form of yoga that is far too aggressive for fibro patients. Look for beginner classes or those that are more focused on gentle stretching. Talk to the instructor about your limitations, and be honest. Don't let yourself be pushed too hard.

Fact

Not all forms of yoga are created equal. Some, such as Iyengar, emphasize precise alignment of the body. Ashtanga yoga is more rigorous and moves rapidly from one pose to another. Kundalini yoga involves chanting, meditation, breathing, and asanas that stimulate the nervous system and release blocked energy. Make sure to choose a yoga class and instructor that together focus on a form that works for you.

Tai Chi

Numerous studies have emerged in recent years touting the health benefits of tai chi, a gentle exercise program derived from the Chinese martial arts. Practitioners do a series of slow deliberate movements, meditation, and deep breathing that are meant to balance the qi, or life energy.

Done regularly, tai chi can improve your muscle tone, balance, agility, and coordination. It can also build strength and improve flexibility. Studies have linked it to stronger bones, less arthritis pain, and even lower blood pressure.

The only downside to tai chi is that some techniques require you to use certain muscles in a way that may be too painful for people with moderate to severe fibromyalgia. Standing on one leg, even for fifteen seconds, may set off cramps or cause a pain flare. It's a good idea to watch a session before trying it to make sure that you are comfortable with the activities involved.

Qi Gong

Qi gong is an ancient body movement developed by the Chinese to improve health, cure disease, and promote longevity. The practice incorporates physical postures with breathing techniques and focused intention. Practitioners may do gentle, rhythmic movements, which can help relieve stress, build stamina, increase vitality, and enhance the immune system.

People who practice qi gong regularly say it helps them remain vital and healthy, even in old age. It also reduces high blood pressure, and promotes better balance, thereby reducing the risk of falling. Qi gong may be done internally, much like meditation with visualizations, or externally, which incorporates movement with meditation. But people with fibromyalgia should steer clear of any form of qi gong that involves physical contact.

Cardiovascular Exercise

The heart-thumping workout of a kickboxing class, a brisk walk, or a long swim are all cardiovascular exercises, activities that strengthen your endurance and heart. When you engage in cardiovascular exercises, you breathe harder, so your lungs are working harder, too. These exercises also improve blood flow, prevent weight gain, and lower blood pressure, triglycerides, and LDL cholesterol, the bad cholesterol. They train your heart to work harder, improving its endurance and overall health. Endurance exercises can minimize depression, reduce stress, and improve sleep. Examples of cardio exercise include jogging, brisk walking, swimming, and aerobics.

For someone in the throes of fibromyalgia, getting a cardiovascular workout might seem too intimidating, especially if you're new to exercise. The thought of even driving to a pool might seem too painful, much less getting in and swimming laps. And indeed, overexertion of any sort could exacerbate your pain and fatigue. But study after study has shown that it's cardiovascular (aerobic) exercise that does the most good for fibro sufferers.

That's why it's important to do cardio exercises and to choose your cardio workout carefully. Avoid high-impact exercises that might exhaust the muscles or cause excess fatigue. Instead, stick with low-impact activities that are less strenuous. Good options include walking, riding a stationary bike, or water aerobics, especially if you can find a pool with warm water. If you prefer stationary biking, be sure to practice good posture with your back straight and your neck upright.

Question

Can I do water exercises if I can't swim?
Absolutely. Swimming is only one way to work out in water. You can also do exercises and movements while standing in shoulder- or chest-high water. For information, contact your local Arthritis Foundation chapter. You can also find information at the Arthritis Foundation Web site on water exercise and arthritis at *www.arthritis.org*.

A Word on Walking

Few exercises can top walking when it comes to safety, convenience, and ease. It requires no special equipment, does not involve a pricey gym membership, and can be done virtually anywhere. You don't even need any special training. All you do need is a good pair of walking shoes. Walking is also unlikely to cause injuries that might deter you from exercising in the future.

If you decide that walking is the best exercise for you, then by all means, give it a try. Always wear a good pair of well-fitting shoes that provide adequate support. Replace old shoes that may be unevenly worn, which can cause an imbalance in your footing and lead to muscle pain.

Start any walk with gentle stretching. When you do start walking, go slowly and resist the urge to walk lengthy distances. Pushing yourself too hard can lead to injuries that interfere with exercising regularly, which is more important than getting a strenuous workout. While you walk, make sure to breathe as normally as possible. To stay safe, walk in well-populated areas or carry a cell phone in case of emergency. If it's hot, carry a water bottle so you can stay hydrated. Finish the walk with a cool-down walk and some gentle stretching.

Strength Training

In general, people with fibromyalgia should avoid strength training. Strength training is far more likely to cause a flare of fibromyalgia than aerobic training, and it should only be done under the supervision of a trainer who is very knowledgeable about fibromyalgia. Otherwise, it can cause far more problems than benefits. In addition, it should not be tried if you have moderate or severe fibro.

When Pain Strikes

Pain is a clear sign that you've overdone it. While most people who exercise work to a level that causes pain, this approach just doesn't work with fibro patients, who have to be much more careful. If you exercise to the point of pain, you can count on feeling pain the next day. Be sure to follow the guidelines discussed above—start low, and go slow. Sometimes even the most careful fibro patient overdoes it. Perhaps you were having a bad day. Or maybe you were coming down with an infection. Maybe you just didn't realize how hard you were working out.

Essential

If you don't like classes, walking, or being at a gym, give exercise videos a try. You can do these any time you like in the privacy of your own home. Best of all, you can do them at your own pace and quit any time you like. Check for videos in your local library or bookstore. You can also order them through organizations such as the National Fibromyalgia Research Association at *www.nfra.net*.

Once pain strikes, it's important to take care of it. If an area feels stiff or sore, give it a gentle massage, or try soaking in a hot bath. If you notice swelling, be careful. It might be a sign of significant tissue injury. Apply a cold pack—a bag of frozen corn or peas will do—to the injured area. If you don't have a history of stomach problems, take ibuprofen or naproxen to lessen pain and reduce the likelihood of spasms or secondary inflammation of the tissue.

You can also prevent pain before a workout by massaging your muscles or wearing elastic supports. Stretching and starting slow to get warmed up are important, too. And avoid working out right after you eat—your body will be diverting blood from your muscles to your intestines, which increases the likelihood of cramps and/or post-workout soreness. After a workout, you can try applying cold to sore muscles for ten to fifteen minutes. The cold can lessen pain and reduce muscle spasms.

Staying Motivated

If it's been a while since you exercised regularly, it might be hard at first to make physical activity a regular part of your routine, especially if you have fibromyalgia. Most of us live very busy lives, and it's easy to abandon plans to exercise in favor of a night out with the girls, a work event, or a shopping excursion. And if you're suffering more pain than usual, it becomes even easier to shrug off a workout. But exercising regularly should be a priority for anyone who has fibromyalgia. Here are ways to help you stick with your exercise program:

- Choose activities you enjoy. Look for activities that spark your interest to improve the odds that you'll keep doing them.
- Write it on your calendar. If you write your exercise commitment down like you would any other appointment, you'll be more apt to stick with it.
- Consider enlisting a workout buddy. Having someone with you will help you pass the time.
- Set specific goals. Set both short- and long-term goals that will give you something to strive for.
- Reward yourself. Buy a new pair of walking shoes, go see a show, or treat yourself to a manicure or, better yet, a massage.

- Spice things up with variety. Avoid boredom by varying your workouts.
- Occupy your mind. Portable music devices help take your mind off the exercise itself; up-tempo is better to energize you for the activity.

Attitude is everything when it comes to staying motivated. If you view yourself as a helpless victim of circumstance, you're less likely to stick with your goals, including your exercise goals. So take steps to stay positive about what you're doing and who you are. Avoid friends who make you feel bad about yourself, and do activities that reinforce your competence.

Make It a Habit

Now that you know why it matters, what to do, and even a little about how to do it, make exercise a habit. Treat it the same way as you do all the other habits in your life, such as brushing your teeth, calling your mom, or watering your garden. Exercising on weekends only or once in a while isn't enough to make difference when it comes to sustaining the improvement.

Brief periods of busyness or excessive pain can be expected for people who have fibromyalgia. Forgive yourself for these temporary disruptions, but then get back on the beat. The key is to keep doing it whenever you can, as often as you can, even if it means doing it in short five- or 10-minute spurts for a while. Try to reinforce your new habit by reading about the health benefits of exercise, surrounding yourself with other people who enjoy exercise, and keeping a journal to remind you of how the activity makes you feel.

Then, just do it! It can take up to six months to build a new habit, but the rewards are well worth it. Besides getting better control of your pain and fatigue, you'll have more energy, more strength, and even more confidence. You may even notice a smaller waistline and better muscle tone. All these factors will contribute to a better quality of life.

Tame the Stress Monster

Getting a handle on stress is critical if you have fibromyalgia. Stress actually makes your pain worse and can make good sleep impossible. Getting it under control can make fibro a little more bearable. In this chapter, we'll take a look at stress, why it's bad, and what you can do about it.

The Stress Response

Everyone has stress. Whether it's the child who's anxious about a test or the adult who's struggling to get along with the in-laws, stress is a normal part of life. It's also not necessarily a bad thing. In small doses, stress can enhance our performance, help us persevere through an emergency, and push us toward higher goals. More important, stress can be essential to our survival. Here's how it works.

Imagine walking alone through a dark park late at night. Suddenly, from behind, you hear footsteps closing in. All senses go into high alert. Your pace quickens, your breathing becomes fast, and your heart begins to race as your body braces itself to defend against the potential attacker.

Meanwhile, several events are taking place inside your body so that you can be prepared to deal with what you sense might be danger. In the brain, the hypothalamus releases corticotropin-releasing hormone (CRH). CRH then triggers the release of norephinephrine, epinephrine—more popularly known as adrenaline—and cortisol, three hormones that work together to help the body brace itself to fight or flee by temporarily improving strength and agility, bolstering concentration and reaction time, and mobilizing reserves of fat and carbohydrates for immediate energy. If the person behind you grabs for your purse, you're braced to fight or to chase him down the street.

Now assume the person walking behind you passes by, and you realize he's simply running to catch a bus. The threat disappears. Your heart rate slows, and you feel calmer. Most of the hormones' levels drop. The exception is cortisol, which continues acting on the brain to halt the production of CRH in order to stop the stress response.

Under these kinds of situations, stress is a necessary defense mechanism that ensures your survival. The problem occurs when stress is chronic, as it often is when you have a chronic illness like fibromyalgia that is tiring, painful, and unpredictable. Other sources might be nightly arguments in a fragile marriage, the threat of job cuts, or even the responsibility of planning a wedding.

Alert

One of the biggest sources of stress is time. Make sure you don't overbook your schedule. Build in get-ready time when you need to get children out the door. Leave a little early if you don't like arriving late. Likewise, bring a book or your latest knitting project, if you think you're going to be held up somewhere.

Living with chronic stress is harmful to your health. It keeps your body in a perpetual state of fight or flight, even when there is nothing to run from and your body isn't moving. As a result, your muscles remain tense, your mind unsettled, and your stomach uneasy. Allowed to linger, chronic stress weakens the immune system, and makes you vulnerable to everything from the common cold to anxiety and depression.

Stress and Fibromyalgia

People who have fibromyalgia deal with a lot more than the stress of constant pain and fatigue. Experts believe that people with FMS actually suffer from a malfunction in the hypothalamic-pituitary-adrenal (HPA) axis, the body's primary communications channel for dealing with stress. Research has shown that people with fibromyalgia have much higher ongoing stress levels than normal people. As a result, they secrete hormones in the HPA axis differently, which can deplete their levels of essential stress hormones, such as cortisol and adrenaline. These reduced levels contribute to the chronic stress and ill feeling that's common among people with fibro.

Stress Aggravates Pain

Virtually any kind of pain is worse when it's accompanied by stress. Premenstrual cramps are more aggravating when you're stressed out at work. A backache is more painful when you're having problems getting along with your spouse. Arthritis typically hurts more when you're dealing with holiday preparations. The same is true for people with fibromyalgia. In fact, stress is one of the triggering factors that can set off a bad flare-up.

Stress Inhibits Sleep

One reason your pain may worsen when you're stressed out is that chronic stress makes it hard to sleep. Your mind is busy dwelling on your lengthy to-do list, your new assignment at work, or the argument you had with your husband. If you have fibromyalgia, you may be fretting about what you can no longer get done or how you're going to handle your pain. As a result, you cannot relax, and so you toss and turn.

Stress Worsens Fibro Fog

When stress is chronic, you lose the ability to concentrate. Your memory falters, and you're not as sharp as you might have been. For people with fibromyalgia who are already vulnerable to fibro fog, stress only makes matters worse. Add sleep deprivation and the side effects of some medications, and you can see how fibro fog can become a serious, debilitating problem. You may find yourself at a loss for words, unable to focus even on simple tasks, and incapable of remembering anything new.

Stress and Diet

Anyone who's ever numbed the stress of a bad experience with a pint of Ben & Jerry's knows it's true: Stress makes us fat. When we're feeling down, most of us are more apt to grab a pint of fudge-brownie ice cream than we are to hit the treadmill.

Question

Why do I eat so poorly when I'm stressed?
Loading up on carbohydrates may do more than make you feel better. Scientists think that fats and sugar may actually help the body silence the stress response. Researchers at the University of California in San Francisco found that after eating sucrose and fats, stressed-out rats showed a decrease in their production of cortisol.

Even without a major catastrophe such as death, divorce, or a move, many of us spend our days fretting and worrying about troubles big and small while sitting in a chair or lying in bed. Problem is, your body doesn't know that you're at a standstill and continues to trigger the stress response, which ratchets up your appetite and tells you to replenish your energy stores. To make matters worse, stress tends to cause cravings for cakes and candy, fats, and carbohydrates that deliver fast energy.

Eating high-fat, high-carb foods while you're under stress may also be a learned behavior, taught by well-meaning relatives who encouraged you to eat a bowl of ice cream when you were feeling sad or gave you cookies after a bad day at school. To top it off, cortisol tends to cause us to deposit fat in our abdomen. In any case, the result is the same—weight gain from overeating due to stress.

Eating poorly is only one unhealthy habit that can crop up during a stressful spell. When you're in the throes of stress, it's easy to let go of healthy habits you've spent years cultivating. Not only are you more likely to grab for a candy bar than an apple, but you're also less likely to exercise, sleep well, and take care of yourself.

If you have fibromyalgia or another chronic condition, you may be less likely to remember your medications, make necessary doctor appointments, and perform the strategies you need to stay well. And if stress evolves into full-blown depression, you may adopt a lackadaisical attitude that can interfere with your efforts to stay healthy.

Controlling Stress

Now that you know all the negative impacts of stress, you understand why it's so important to take control of it. Left to linger, uncontrolled stress influences almost every aspect of your well-being and takes a negative toll on your health.

Truth is, you will always have stressors in your life. Whether it's a job you hate, a wedding you have to plan, or a long commute to cope with, stress is an inevitable part of our existence. But stress doesn't just come from events that occur. Stress is also the result of how you perceive an event. For instance, you might find it stressful to sit through a traffic jam. But your best friend might view it as an opportunity to hear a radio talk show she enjoys. Shifting your thinking to a less stressful mindset, then, can play a key role in taking control of stress. Taking charge of stress then must take place on three levels:

- First, you must try to reduce the numbers of events that potentially stress you out. While you certainly can't control every aspect of your life, you can minimize those that cause you undue anxiety.
- Second, practice altering your perspective of troubling events. Maybe you can't give your boss a personality makeover, but you can change the way you think of her.
- Finally, make time to relax in order to counter the effects of stress. If stress is truly inevitable, then you need strategies that keep it in check.

Attacking stress on all three levels will help you reduce it and prevent your fibro symptoms from worsening. Although nothing can ever completely eliminate stress, the following strategies can help buffer you from it.

 ## Fact

Research shows that stress in the workplace is more strongly associated with health complaints than any other stressor, including financial problems or family troubles. According to the National Institute for Occupational Safety and Health, the primary cause of workplace stress is working conditions, but the personal characteristics and circumstances of the workers also plays a role.

Scale Back

When you have a chronic condition like fibromyalgia, it's important to prioritize and do those things that matter most. This goes back to what we've said before about setting priorities, delegating, and learning to pace yourself. Attempting to do it all or trying to do too much will result in stress, especially when you find that you can no longer do all that you once did. By cutting back on your activities, workload, and responsibilities, you'll find you're less stressed and better able to endure the challenges of fibromyalgia.

Sleep If Possible

A good night's rest is one of the most potent weapons against stress. When you're rested, you're better able to withstand life's little annoyances—the surly sales clerk, the long lines, the unexpected flat tire—than you are when you're tired. So while getting a good night's sleep might seem impossible with fibromyalgia, it's important to try to adopt strategies that can enhance your sleep. That means making sleep a priority, going to bed on a schedule, and avoiding activities and substances that interfere with sleep.

Practice Relaxation

Making time to relax can make a world of difference in how you feel. It's a chance for you to pause, rejuvenate, and recharge—mentally, physically, even emotionally. Unfortunately, relaxation falls to the bottom of the priority list when you're trying to keep up with everything else on your to-do list. But when you have fibromyalgia, it's important to put relaxation back at the top of your priorities. Think of it as a special time for you. Here are some ways to relax throughout your day:

- Take a break with a cup of hot herbal tea.
- During the day, take a short walk with a friend.
- Consider learning meditation.
- Make time to stretch every hour or two.
- Call a friend who makes you laugh.

Banish Negative Self-Talk

Most of us have a voice inside our head that offers running commentary on how we're doing in our lives. A positive voice can work wonders toward helping you achieve your goals. That voice might tell you, "You're doing great!" or "They really like you." But some people are prone to hearing negative self-talk that can cause unwarranted stress and anxiety.

People who have fibromyalgia may be especially vulnerable when they're still trying to get a handle on their condition. Here are a few examples of this type of negative self-talk:

- "I'll never live normally again."
- "I can't possibly get it done."
- "It's all my fault."
- "I can never do it as well as _____ does."
- "I should be doing _____."

When you're trying to control stress, it's important to banish these kinds of negative, all-or-nothing thoughts. Overgeneralizing and setting impossible standards with "should" statements won't help either. You also need to get away from blaming yourself, comparing yourself to others, and setting yourself up for failure by taking on an impossibly long list of chores. So instead of the above statements, try telling yourself some of the following:

- "I may not be well, but I'll do my best."
- "I'll do what I can and do the rest another time."
- "Getting sick can happen to anyone."
- "_____ may do better at this, but it doesn't really matter."
- "I need to take care of my health first."

Eat Well

It's tempting to dive into a bowl of macaroni and cheese when we're feeling stressed out. Traditional comfort foods are often associated with making us feel safe and secure. But in reality, these foods can make us feel lethargic. In the long run, too much of these soothing, high-fat foods can promote weight gain. Instead, when you're stressed, you should focus on eating nutritious foods, such as fruits and vegetables, which can help bolster an immune system already taxed by stress. If you prefer carbohydrates, strive to eat the complex kind, such as whole-grain breads, pastas, and cereals. Also include low-fat sources of protein in your diet, such as fish, lean beef, turkey, and tofu. Finally, drink plenty of water.

At the same time, you need to avoid foods that contain caffeine, sugar, fat, and salt, which exacerbate the symptoms of stress, especially if eaten in large quantities. These foods can also cause weight gain. Also beware of consuming too much alcohol, especially if you've had a substance abuse problem in the past. In large amounts, alcohol will compound your stress and prevent you from dealing effectively with your fibromyalgia.

Alert

Some people react to stress by undereating, perhaps forgetting to eat or not eating enough. To enhance your appetite, make meal-times relaxed and pleasant. Avoid dealing with unpleasant topics before and during meals. Eat with family or friends who may help relax you. If possible, take a short walk before a meal to stimulate the appetite. Finally, stock the house with your favorite healthy foods.

Exercise

When you're in a perpetual state of fight or flight, your body actually wants activity. Moving your body will help release some of the pent-up energy that's been stored in the event of a real emergency. It also releases feel-good endorphins that help produce the relaxation response.

So make regular exercise a priority. Don't get in the habit of skipping it when you're too busy or too tired. That's when you're most likely to be stressed and in need of a good workout. Regular activity will reduce stress, improve function, and help you sleep better at night.

Treat Yourself Well

Too often, we race through life trying to attend to all our responsibilities and obligations—most often to other people. What you should do instead is something special for yourself every day. Whether it's renting a beloved movie, getting a manicure, or spending time with a special friend, don't shy away from indulgences, even when you're not feeling your best. In fact, sometimes a little self-soothing is just what you need to distract you from your pain and fatigue. That's what Amy learned to do when her pain got bad.

During a fibro flare, Amy learned she had to stop, rest, and enjoy some quiet fun. She kept a ready stack of funny movies and indulged in childhood activities like coloring, blowing bubbles, and playing with Play Dough. Sometimes, she just sat and read magazines or books. The respites helped her get through her toughest moments.

Surrender When Necessary

Everyone knows about those unexpected fiascos that interrupt our best laid plans—the mechanic who forgot to order the must-have part, the traffic accident that blocked up the road, and the computer crash that annihilated your newest files. Rather than fume about it, ask yourself, "Is there really anything I can do about this?" Chances are good that there's nothing you can do.

Once you realize that these incidents are beyond your control, go into planning mode and think about what you can do instead. Maybe you can ask the mechanic to fix something else while you're there. Perhaps you can listen to your favorite CD until the accident clears up. Maybe a tech specialist can help you retrieve at least some of the work you lost. In some cases, you might simply have to chalk up the annoyance to a real bummer and move on. Remind yourself that letting it go is better for your health.

Breathe Deeply

We take our breaths for granted, but in fact, breathing is a wonderful tool for relaxation, one that also eliminates toxins and naturally lowers blood pressure and heart rate. When you stop to breathe, it helps shift your focus on to something other than the stressor at hand.

If you suffer from shortness of breath, try breathing through pursed lips. The technique slows the pace of your breathing and makes each breath more effective. Start by relaxing your shoulder and neck muscles. Then inhale slowly through your nose for two counts, making sure not to breathe too deeply. Next, pucker as if you were going to whistle or blow out a candle. Exhale slowly and gently through pursed lips as you count to four. The technique will relax you and improve your breathing pattern.

Get Organized

Chaos may signal creativity for some people, but in the life of someone with a chronic illness that's so unpredictable, unfettered messes can be stressful. Cluttered rooms, messy work places, and disorganized papers can make it hard to function or think clearly. In a bedroom, it can even disrupt sleep.

Trying to locate an important file is the last thing you want to deal with when you're living with fibromyalgia. Next time you have a good day, devote some time to cleaning out clutter and organizing stuff. Don't try to organize the entire house at once. Just do a single drawer, closet, or area of a room at a time. Your body will thank you later.

Pinpoint Big Stressors

Often, people go about their day putting out one fire after another or moving from task to task. That's fine when you're feeling well. But when you're not, it helps to figure out exactly what issues stress you most and to devise strategies in advance for dealing with them.

Essential

Not sure what stresses you out? Try keeping a stress journal. Record the day, the time, and any incidents that increase your anxiety. After a while, you'll see a pattern and be better able to see what has you stressed out. In a few weeks, you can compile a list and rank them by severity. Use the information to help you develop coping strategies.

If it's being late for work, then maybe you need to do more preparations at night. If it's the stream of bills that you can't pay, maybe you should meet with a financial counselor. If it's low energy on a busy day, then maybe you should create a list of things you can do another time. The idea is to become aware of your stress triggers and to effectively nip them in the bud.

Assume Control

When you're not feeling well, it's easy to displace responsibilities on to other people. In some cases, it's essential to delegate certain tasks, such as preparing dinner, cleaning the house, or paying bills. But the big picture—namely all aspects of your health and well-being—should be in your hands. You should pick and choose the doctors you want, the activities you do, and the friends that surround you. By taking charge, you'll feel much more confident and in charge. And that alone can help you feel less stressed when life does throw you a curve ball.

Changing Your Thinking

A great deal of stress can be caused by the way you perceive the events in your life, not what's actually happening. For instance, planning a birthday party for your child can be enormously stressful for one mother, while another may find it a delightful pleasure. Changing the way you perceive things isn't easy and requires constant practice. Many of these thought processes are built up over a lifetime and then become ingrained as habits, automatic responses—often emotional—to what is going on around you. Sometimes, it takes the professional counseling of a trained therapist to change the way you think. This type of therapy is known as cognitive behavioral therapy.

But that doesn't mean you can't work at diminishing negative thoughts on your own. According to MindTools.com, a Web site devoted to helping people excel in their careers, the first step is to cultivate greater awareness of your thoughts and thought patterns. What kinds of events trigger these negative thoughts? Who are the people involved? Next, you need to apply rational thinking and facts to your thoughts. Consider this your reality check. Finally, you need to come up with affirmations that counter the negative thinking with positive thoughts.

For instance, let's assume you are always worried that your boss doesn't like the work you're doing. When he doesn't greet you in the morning, you take it as a sure-fire sign that he's displeased with your latest assignment. But weeks go by, and he says nothing. Instead, he gives you another challenging task to take on.

Alert

It's normal to worry about things like an upcoming presentation or a big party you're throwing. But constant worry over routine everyday events may be an indication of generalized anxiety disorder (GAD), especially when the worry becomes chronic. Fortunately, GAD can be treated with medications or therapy. But untreated, GAD can lead to full-blown depression.

In this case, the negative thinking stems from worries about job performance. For a more rational look at the situation, you need to ask yourself a few rational questions. Did I give it my best? Was I well prepared? Could I have really done any better? Then, consider the facts. If your boss was truly displeased, wouldn't he have said something? And why would he be giving you another plum assignment? Finally, you should adopt some new thoughts to change the old negative ones. Some good ones might include, "I always do my best. I am always well prepared. I have a history of doing well at my work."

Stress-Free Relationships

One of the greatest sources of stress comes from the people we know, sometimes even the ones we love. Think of the mother who can't resist nagging, the spouse who refuses to do his share of chores, or the friend who can never keep her lunch plans with you. Annoying, right? Then add in those people that we're forced to deal with—the moody boss, the nosy neighbor, or the hostile sales clerk. Just navigating the land mine of human relations can be a major source of stress.

For most of us, it's impossible to eliminate all the people in our lives who stress us out. But now that you have fibromyalgia, you might need to mend, tweak, or, in some cases, terminate some of these relationships so that you feel less stress. In some cases, you might need to confront the problem. Talk things over with people who bother you. Don't let bad feelings fester so that you're left feeling angry or annoyed. On some matters, you might be able to reach a compromise or resolution.

When it comes to people you can't avoid, you might have to change the way you relate to them. If your sister drives you crazy, restrict your communication to e-mail and the occasional phone call. If your father-in-law bothers you at family gatherings, you might just have to avoid him as much as possible. In some cases, you might need to consider ending your energy-sapping relationships. Some people are simply not worth the trouble and stress they cause. Ask yourself, "What am I really getting out of this relationship?" If the relationship is no longer rewarding and possibly even hurtful, then maybe it's time to end it.

Remember, working on the relationships in your life that cause stress might be the toughest challenge of all. In fact, it might cause you some stress while you're in the process. But don't be afraid to speak up and make your needs heard. Your number-one priority now is to take care of your health. Consider the case of Janet.

> When Janet first got sick, many friends didn't understand the pain she was experiencing. Even her family members didn't grasp the extent of her challenges. Over time, some of Janet's friends stopped calling her, and Janet didn't bother to try and find them. Instead, she found new friends, especially at her yoga class, who understood her circumstances. "I'm a major believer in keeping the energy around you positive," she says. "My mantra is: remove all toxic things and toxic people."

Although Janet was effectively able to rid her life of toxic people, she still couldn't quite get away from family members who don't believe she has anything wrong with her. With them, she has simply chosen to limit her contact and instead spends her time with friends who do understand and a husband and a daughter whom she adores.

CHAPTER 15

Managing
Difficult Emotions

Even the most stoic person experiences a range of emotions with a chronic illness like fibromyalgia. You may feel sad, even depressed, over the chronic pain. You may be angry about being sick. And you may feel frustrated that you even have fibromyalgia if you've always tried to stay healthy. The key to handling emotions is to accept the way you feel, deal with the emotions, and then make sure that they don't interfere with your ability to take care of yourself.

Mourning Your Condition

Feeling more than a little blue is common when you're sick, especially when it's a chronic illness like fibromyalgia, which has no cure. After all, FMS impacts so many aspects of your life, from your ability to sleep to the skills you need to perform your job. In some people, sadness can evolve into depression, a serious mental illness that warrants medical attention. Left untreated, depression can ravage your family life, career, and relationships, causing enormous pain and suffering.

Not surprisingly, people with fibro are more vulnerable to depression than the average healthy adult—studies have shown that about a third of them are depressed at any point in time. Others who are able to escape the grips of depression still battle periodic bouts of overwhelming sadness. You may feel sad because you can no longer move around as easily. You may feel sad because the fatigue limits what you can do in a day. You may even grieve because you have lost a part of yourself to a baffling medical condition.

It's perfectly normal to go through periods of intense sadness and mourning. Allowing yourself the time and space to grieve will help you get past it. It will also enable you to start taking the steps you need to manage your fibromyalgia. In the meantime, your sadness may be masked by other emotions.

Denial

Perhaps you know someone who has fibromyalgia, or you've read about the disease. When you learn that it's happening to you, you simply can't believe it. You go looking for all the reasons why it can't be.

Some people react to learning they have fibromyalgia with disbelief and denial. In the short term, denial can be positive. Denying you have fibro gives you a chance to recoup. It buys you time while you adjust to the idea of having a medical condition. It also allows you to keep hoping that nothing is really wrong until you learn to accept your situation. But if you remain in denial too long, it can interfere with your ability to face reality and take care of yourself.

Anger

It's normal to feel angry about having fibromyalgia. After all, you did nothing to bring on this condition. In fact, you may have even been the pillar of good health, someone who didn't smoke or drink, ate well, and exercised regularly.

Now that you've been diagnosed with a chronic disease that causes immense pain and fatigue, you're furious and possibly asking, "Why me?" You're angry that doctors ignore you, that friends don't believe you, and that doing anything takes enormous effort. Compounding your rage is the unpredictability of fibromyalgia, making it hard for you to plan anything.

Getting over your anger isn't easy and may take time. But not getting rid of it can take a toll on your health. Anger can worsen your sleep, exacerbate your pain, and interfere with your ability to take care of yourself. It also saps your already compromised energy levels.

That's why it's important to acknowledge your anger, use it to motivate you to make positive change, express it in positive ways, and then move on. Here are some ways to do that:

- Get to the root of your anger. Are you mad because you can't do all the things you used to do? That you're overwhelmed with fatigue? That you feel helpless? Identify the cause of your anger, and try to work on that.
- Talk it out. Whether it's a close friend or a professional counselor, venting your anger can help reduce it. Your friend or counselor may be able to see your situation from a different perspective and help you overcome your anger.
- Get real. Rather than dwell on what you used to do, create new expectations of yourself. By keeping your expectations realistic and attainable, you'll build your sense of competence and rein in frustration.
- Channel your anger into action. Rather than devoting too much energy to feeling mad, try putting that energy toward positive action. Fed up that you can't cook the way you used to? Think of it as a challenge to find simpler recipes.
- Beware the dark side of anger. If not expressed constructively, anger can come out as irritability toward your family, friends, and colleagues. This can cost you valued, supportive relationships. So when you do express anger, do so constructively, not destructively.

Experts have long suspected a link between anger and depression and heart disease, but these emotions may actually spur biological changes in the body. A study published in 2004 found that people who were angry and had more severe depressive symptoms—separately and in combination with hostility—had higher levels of C-reactive protein, a substance in the body released in response to stress and infection that has been linked to heart disease.

Guilt

Some people may blame themselves for "getting" fibromyalgia. You may dwell on the things you could have done differently that could have prevented fibromyalgia. For some people—especially if your self-esteem is already fragile—having fibromyalgia may be an indication of personal failure or fault. Many FMS patients often feel guilty about things they think they should accomplish that they no longer can, especially when it comes to parenting responsibilities.

Guilt can become a major obstacle if you wallow in it. It can get in the way of taking care of yourself, especially if you think you're impinging on others by asking for their support or that you don't think you deserve proper treatment. When you're sick with a chronic condition, there's no room for destructive emotions like guilt. Acknowledge these bad feelings, but then move on. Remember: You do deserve the extra care and attention, and you did absolutely nothing to deserve your illness.

Fear

It's completely normal to feel fearful and anxious in the face of a chronic condition that fluctuates. You may be wondering if you'll ever be well again. The possibility that you won't recover can make you extremely frightened about your future. You may fear losing your job, your friends, your family, or your lifestyle.

But too much fear can worsen your symptoms. It can cause muscle tension, stomach pain, and a racing heart. In turn, you may notice that your pain is worse and that getting sleep is even more difficult. The resulting fatigue will only exacerbate your symptoms. If your fears become overwhelming, they can put you on edge even on days when you feel good. You may routinely feel helpless and unable to control your fibro.

Fear can become a vicious cycle. The more you worry, the more you find to worry about, and the more little problems escalate into big problems. The fear then builds, causing stress that only makes your fibromyalgia worse. Taming your fear is important. Here are some suggestions from the Web site CFIDS & Fibromyalgia Self-Help, *www.cfidsselfhelp.org*:

- Solve your problems. If it's a practical matter that has you anxious, solving it can reduce your worry and boost your confidence.
- Practice stress reduction. Taking action against stress can create a calming effect that silences your worrying, too.
- Change your thinking. Rather than think in catastrophic terms, like, "I'll never get through this," tell yourself things like, "This is not as bad as it seems."
- Connect with others. Whether it's volunteer work or taking a class, getting involved in something larger than yourself counteracts and distracts you from your own worries.
- Exercise. Not only is activity good for your body, but it is also relaxing and distracting.
- Do something pleasurable. Read a good book, listen to music, or call a friend. Enjoyable activities can help change your mood and shift your focus.
- Share your worries. Discuss your concerns with a trusted friend or relative. It will make your worries less scary.

If fear and anxiety begin to take over your life, get professional help. Your doctor may be able to prescribe medications to help reduce your anxiety.

Loneliness

When you're sick, it often feels as if no one could possibly feel as bad as you do. Truth is, millions of people suffer from fibromyalgia, so you're far from alone. But knowing that doesn't always help when you're in the grips of severe pain and no one around you seems to understand.

In reality, you may become somewhat isolated when you're first dealing with fibromyalgia. Friends who don't know how to help may back away. You may be in too much pain to socialize. Family members may be at loss as to how to help.

Try to accept your isolation as a temporary phase. Then, as you gradually come to terms with having FMS, focus on broadening your social experiences. Look for support groups where you might meet others with fibromyalgia. Ask your physician for information about classes that can help you. Go online to Web sites of fibro organizations that have bulletin boards where you can share with others. Staying in touch with the world will minimize loneliness.

 Alert

Spouses of people who have fibromyalgia are more vulnerable to loneliness, depression, and stress than those whose partners are well, according to one study. So make sure your partner takes steps to stay well, too. Encourage him or her to exercise, practice relaxation, and remain socially engaged.

Coping with Emotions

Most people faced with a serious illness will ride an emotional roller coaster. But the timing of your emotions will vary depending on your individual circumstances. For instance, if it took a long time for you to get diagnosed, you might feel relief at first, even joy, then move on to anger and feelings of isolation later on. Or if you already suffer from low self-esteem, you may feel worthless and guilty right at the start. Those who are prone to stress may be bitter and angry, without feeling sadness.

Some people's emotions follow the same course as the ones outlined by Elisabeth Kubler-Ross and her research on the stages of grief. In her book *On Death and Dying*, Kubler-Ross identified five stages experienced by a patient diagnosed with a terminal disease: denial, anger, bargaining, depression, and sadness. Although fibromyalgia is not a deadly disease, the disappointment that can come with having it will almost certainly trigger a grieving process.

Essential

Resilience—the ability to survive hardship—can help you persevere through life's most difficult circumstances. The American Psychological Association offers an online brochure called "The Road to Resilience" that can help anyone build resilience. For information, check out the Web site at the APA Help Center (*www.helping.apa.org*).

In any case, powerful emotions are part of getting diagnosed with a chronic illness. Whatever path your emotions take, it's important not to let them overwhelm you and prevent you from getting the care you need. There are several strategies that can help make you more resilient.

Control Issues

Learning to let go of things you can't control is important for people who have fibromyalgia, not just in terms of their health but in terms of their lives. The only thing you can do is to stop worrying about things you can't control. Try to accept that fibro flares are often unpredictable, that the effects of a medication are often a mystery, and that your day-to-day symptoms will vary. Instead, focus on the moment. That's what Regina does to survive her fibro pain.

As an actress, Regina was trained to work with the magic of the moment. Having lived with fibromyalgia for almost two years now, Regina applies that lesson to her fibromyalgia. So even when she's hurting, she focuses on what else is happening at the moment, which is often more monumental and significant than the pain in her body. "It's a day-to-day process," she says. "I listen to my body, but refuse to be enslaved by it. I don't believe that my body is me. I believe my mind and heart is me, and that helps free me from the pain."

 ## Alert

Do not compare yourself to others. Trying to keep up with other people, especially those who don't have a chronic illness, will set you up for distressing emotions, such as frustration, anger, and sadness. It also distracts you from living life in the moment and forces you to dwell on what should have, could have, or would have been— thoughts that will surely cause despair.

Rather than worry about things you did wrong or the future of your health, put your energies into the present, into the very moment. Learn how much you can do without flaring your fibro. Exercise. Stretch. Work on developing a positive attitude. Do affirmations. Write in a journal. Eat properly. Fretting about what's done or what's to come can cause worry and anxiety that will only worsen your symptoms.

Be Realistic

Being unrealistic when you have fibromyalgia only sets you up for disappointment, anger, and frustration. When it happens over and over again, you put yourself at risk for sadness. Keep your plans within reason and certainly within reach. Ask yourself if you can really accomplish what you're planning. For instance, you may have been able to wash and fold three loads of laundry when you were healthy. But now that you have fibromyalgia, it might be more realistic to do one load at a time.

When you're realistic, you also know to accept your limitations. You know you can't hike the way you did before or entertain guests the way you once did. Accept these new developments and look for alternative ways to exercise or entertain. Maybe you can still take slow, easy walks in the neighborhood or host a small group for morning coffee.

Get Positive

Positive thinking can make a world of difference in how you feel emotionally—and physically. While it's impossible for you to think your way out of your illness, the way you think can impact the severity of your symptoms. The more positive you are, the less severe your symptoms will be.

Question

What if I'm a born pessimist?
There's no such thing, according to experts, who say that pessimism and optimism are attitudes you learn. People develop these attitudes in childhood, typically from our parents. Once ingrained, these attitudes can be hard to change. But if you want to change your attitude—and desire is the first step in any change—start by changing the way you think. Having faith that you can change will help spur the process, which can take weeks, even months.

Of course, positive thinking isn't easy when you're feeling so bad. And for some people, who are naturally more cynical and pessimistic, thinking positively doesn't always come naturally. The good news is that you can learn to reframe your thoughts by first recognizing negative thinking and thought patterns, then challenging them with new and positive ideas. According to Dennis C. Turk, director of the Fibromyalgia Research Center and Professor of Anesthesiology and Pain Research at the University of Washington School of Medicine in Seattle, the ways of negative thinking described in the following sections are the most common.

Blaming

Some people mistakenly blame the pain they feel on someone else or on themselves. Excessive self-blame can lead to depression.

"Should" Statements

Should statements suggest that you were weak or stupid for something you did or felt. Examples include, "I should feel better than this," or "I shouldn't have taken that walk."

Polarized Thinking

This type of thinking involves absolutes and uses words such as "every," "none," "never," "always," "everybody," and "anybody." By over-generalizing, you implicitly reinforce the belief that your efforts have failed.

Catastrophizing

Imagining the worst outcome and then reacting as if it's coming true can compound your anxiety. Examples include what-ifs, such as "What if my FM never gets better? What if my spouse leaves me? What if I never work again?"

Control Fallacies

This type of thinking gives another person total power over the fate of others. Thinking that "My family can't function without me," or "My doctor is the only one who can help me" are examples of control fallacies.

Emotional Reasoning

Allowing your emotions to rule reality means operating on the assumption that what you feel is the truth. So if you feel as if you're on the verge of a flare-up, then you will certainly have one tomorrow. Your emotions overwhelm your ability to reason.

Filtering

Focusing only on the negative can obscure something positive that might have occurred or been said. You may choose to remember only those things that support your angry feelings.

Entitlement Fallacy

Some people think that life owes them a pain-free existence. As a result, they feel cheated and focus on the injustice of being sick.

Once you recognize the types of negative thoughts that plague your mind, try to find alternative ways of thinking. Devise new statements and thought patterns that counter the negative ones. Be patient as you work toward change. It will take time to transform your thinking.

Learn to Communicate Effectively

Some people bottle up their feelings. Others send the wrong messages. Still others talk incessantly to the point where their message is lost. But when you have a chronic illness like fibromyalgia, you need to communicate clearly and effectively with everyone around you, from your spouse and your children to your doctors and health-care team.

Effective communication means speaking up and making your needs known. Don't expect that your spouse automatically knows when you're feeling bad or that your friend can tell when you're asking for her help. Tell them. That's how Christina finally got some much-needed child-care assistance from friends.

> Christina had two young kids and a husband who traveled all the time for his job. She also had fibromyalgia. Having the kids around the clock became exhausting until she finally suggested to a friend that they take turns swapping babysitting. The kids had a play date, and the moms got a break. Soon the babysitting swap was a weekly routine. "Now, I tell everyone with fibromyalgia to ask for help," Christina says.

When you do speak up, do it in a way that isn't offensive and abrasive. For instance, announcing to your husband that he never helps around the house is not exactly going to inspire his assistance.

But if you tell him that you'd like it if he could clean the bathrooms this weekend, you're more apt to get the help you want.

Essential

While you're busy trying to communicate your needs, don't forget to be a good listener, too, especially with close family members like your spouse and children. Fibromyalgia can affect everyone in the household, so be ready with open ears to hear what others are worried about.

Need Help?

If you've tried to take control of difficult emotions and still find yourself overwhelmed, it might be time to get help from a mental-health professional. Talking to a professional counselor can sometimes help you overcome the difficulties you have managing your feelings. A therapist can also help you devise strategies to overcome destructive emotions.

Reaching Acceptance

Think of acceptance as the emotional nirvana, when you're no longer bogged down with anger, frustration, and loneliness, when the focus in your life finally shifts to taking care of your health. Don't mistake acceptance for resignation. Acceptance means understanding that your life is now different, but that you can still live a full and purposeful existence.

When you are emotionally ready to accept fibromyalgia, take some time to re-evaluate your life and your lifestyle. Now that your energy and physical abilities are limited, you will have to find new activities to pursue that still spark your passion. You will also have to learn to let certain things go, possibly things you enjoyed in the past. You may even need to launch a new career. Achieving acceptance can also help you figure out what matters most and where you really want to spend your time and limited energy. In the process, you may find new hobbies, develop new friendships, and cultivate new interests that rejuvenate you.

Staying Happy

In this new stage of acceptance, you will feel less encumbered by unpleasant emotions. It isn't that you won't have days when you're angry, sad, or frustrated. These negative emotions are a part of life. But with acceptance comes a greater measure of happiness; you'll feel a sense of moving out of the misery and getting on with your life.

For some people with fibromyalgia, it isn't easy to feel happy. After all, you've lost the ability to do things you enjoy. Your body is wracked with pain. Sleep is elusive, and your days are a foggy blur. On top of it, you're dealing with an endless number of visits to doctors, trying to keep track of numerous medications, and fretting about the course of your illness.

While maintaining a positive outlook isn't easy, it's important to your health. Feeling happy can strengthen your immune system and ensure that you will engage in healthy behaviors that can alleviate your symptoms. Here's how you stay positive when your body feels lousy:

- Steer clear of negative thinking. Look for ways to reframe an event and modify the way you view it.
- Seek out the spiritual. Whether it's organized religion or individual spirituality, putting your faith in a higher power can help you overcome any rough spots you encounter.
- Reach out to others. It's impossible to handle the emotional rigors of illness alone, so spend time with people you care about.
- Try to do something you enjoy every day. Read a book. Go outside and take a walk. Listen to music you enjoy. Giving attention to life's pleasurable experiences will counteract the negative emotions you feel.

The way you choose to pursue happiness is up to you. The key is to do it, even if it doesn't come easily. But when you find yourself immersed in a good book, chuckling through a funny movie, or sharing good conversation with a friend, you'll know that you've achieved happiness, in spite of your pain.

CHAPTER 16

The Mind-Body Connection

One of the most powerful tools in your arsenal against fibromyalgia resides within you. It's your brain, the very organ that is transmitting the pain signals wreaking havoc on your body. Learning to use your mind to control the symptoms of fibromyalgia is a powerful skill, a remarkable defense against the ravages of fibro. In this chapter, we'll show you several ways that you can tap into this extraordinary weapon.

The Power of the Mind

The mind. The body. The spirit. Some say all three are inextricably linked in a complex interweave that plays out in our health and well-being. Think of all the times you were overwhelmed by a stressful event, only to get sick with a cold. Or how you became ill while struggling to overcome the grief of a death in the family. Consider how your bodily aches and pains can make you unhappy and irritable.

 Fact

Adults with long-term musculoskeletal pain were almost twice as likely to use mind-body treatments and prayer than those without. But men were less likely than women to do so. In addition, people who had more than a high school education were more likely to try these therapies than those who went to high school only.

But as anyone who has ever tried meditation or another mind-body technique knows, the mind can also have a positive impact on how you feel. Think of how images of a recent vacation with friends can wipe out the headaches of a stressful job, or how taking deep breaths can ease your anger. Recall those times in the dentist's chair when a happy memory momentarily erased the pain of the drill.

Meditation

In a world that bustles around all day, every day, making time to sit still and breathe seems counterintuitive—and certainly counterproductive. But meditation is one of the oldest and most effective ways to reduce stress, ease anxiety, and tame your muscle pain. Meditating can also enhance immunity, improve sleep, and reduce depression.

Meditation comes in many different forms, including transcendental, mindfulness, and Buddhist. Some may involve movement, such as yoga. Others require sitting without movement. Still others involve going through day-to-day routines in a more mindful manner. All types of meditation, however, have one goal: to silence the busy mind and to direct all attention to a single healing entity such as the breath, a mantra, or image. In a quiet state of meditation, your mind is in the present, not contemplating the past or the future.

For people who have fibromyalgia, meditation can induce a state of calm that lessens the pain. It can also help you assume more control of your condition. Andrea, who has fibromyalgia, credits her improved health entirely to her meditation practice.

> For years, Andrea was popping ibuprofen and acetaminophen in a futile attempt to silence her fibro pain. She tried different exercises and became a vegan. But she credits her gradual recovery to meditation, a practice she began to cultivate five years ago. Gradually, she built up her practice to sitting twice a day, forty-five minutes at a time.
>
> Although she still has flares and experiences pain, Andrea has become more adroit at coping with it. "It's not that the pain has

lessened," she says. "It's that I'm more in touch with how the sensations actually feel rather than the thoughts about them. I used to think, 'Oh my gosh, this is killing me. What am I going to do?' When I stopped freaking out, I realized that the actual sensations are bearable."

Anyone can learn to meditate. It's easy because it doesn't require any special skills, equipment, or clothing. On the other hand, meditation can be extremely difficult, especially if you aren't comfortable with the idea of sitting still. Some people find it easier to meditate in the company of others. For them, a class might be a good idea. But others prefer to meditate alone. Here's how you can give it a try:

1. Find a quiet place in your home where you can sit uninterrupted.
2. Sit in a comfortable position. You might prefer sitting in a chair or against a wall, or simply cross-legged on the floor. However you sit, keep your spine straight.
3. Begin by closing your eyes and gently breathing.
4. Pay attention to your breath as it comes in and goes out.
5. Do your best to focus only on your breathing. If thoughts do arise, acknowledge them, then go back to your breath.
6. If it helps, say a mantra, like "Om," "Love," or "Serenity" or a phrase such as "All is well."
7. Start slowly by meditating for just a few minutes, then build up gradually to longer periods of meditation.

The goal of meditation is to simply be and not do. You want to quiet the mind of its constant chatter. Like anything new, this may seem difficult at first. But with practice, it will become easier.

Hypnosis

When you think of hypnosis, you probably think of the magician who puts an audience member into a trance, then convinces him to do something out of the ordinary. In reality, however, people fall into a hypnotic trance on a regular basis—when they're spellbound by a captivating movie, engrossed in a riveting mystery, or absorbed in a fantasy-filled daydream.

Hypnotherapy, on the other hand, is a treatment that has been used to help smokers quit smoking, insomniacs start sleeping, and people with anxiety overcome their fears. Studies show that hypnotherapy has strong potential for relieving pain, which makes it a likely therapy for fibromyalgia. Some people also practice self-hypnosis.

Essential

Don't worry. Hypnotherapy won't make you vulnerable to bizarre behaviors or the whims of an unscrupulous hypnotist. In fact, you have control the whole time when you're hypnotized.

Contrary to what you see in a magic show, people under hypnosis have complete control of their minds. In fact, the brain is actually more alert and active under hypnosis, even if you feel as if you're dozing off to sleep. The key to using hypnosis as a treatment is to channel that brain activity into your healing.

To find a qualified therapist, start by asking your health-care practitioners or trusted friends for a referral. Choose one who is certified. You can also learn self-hypnosis on your own with the help of books and tapes.

During a hypnotherapy session, you may be asked to sit or lie down. The therapist will make sure you are comfortable and then guide you into a hypnotic state of mind. Some may play soft music. Others may simply talk. The therapist may touch you on your neck, forehead, or wrist to see if you are in a relaxed state, but otherwise, there is no physical contact.

As you enter into a hypnotic trance, your body becomes totally relaxed, your thinking highly focused. While in a trance, the therapist will talk to you about your pain or other symptoms and behaviors you'd like to change. For instance, the therapist may suggest that your pain is subsiding, that your fatigue is diminished. In your hypnotic state, your mind is open to suggestion, and you adopt these thoughts as your own.

Hypnotherapy uses a combination of relaxation and visualization to change thought patterns, emotions, and behaviors. If you frequently respond to your pain with fear and anxiety, hypnosis can train you to modify those thoughts so that you are less reactive and calmer during a flare-up.

Biofeedback

A thermometer. A mirror. A blood-pressure monitor. All these devices are tools that could be considered biofeedback, instruments that provide information about your health that inspire you to improve your well-being. Biofeedback in the more traditional sense involves the use of special equipment to first measure physiological function and then train the patient's mind to respond in a way that promotes healing and better health. Biofeedback has been used for numerous health problems, such as TMJ, stress, and chronic headaches. In people who have fibromyalgia, biofeedback can turn down a stress system that is turned up way too high. It can also help relax tight muscles, which in turn can lessen your pain and fatigue.

Alert

Some companies sell biofeedback equipment for home use. They may also be called neurofeedback. But not all of them work properly or are worth the money. Talk to your doctor before making a purchase.

During biofeedback, you are attached to an electronic monitor that measures bodily functions, such as your brain waves, skin temperature, and blood pressure. While you're hooked up, you will practice relaxation techniques that alter these body functions so that you can increase body temperature, reduce blood pressure, and calm excited brain waves. You will see these changes on the monitor and come to understand which states of mind have what effect on the body. You will also learn how you feel when your blood pressure slows, your body temperature goes up, and brain waves calm down.

With practice, biofeedback will empower you to control bodily functions and lessen your symptoms. The number of sessions you require will vary, depending on the severity of your symptoms and how quickly you learn to train your body. For more information, and to find a qualified biofeedback counselor in your area, check out the Biofeedback Certification Institute of America, online at *www.bcia.org*.

Guided Imagery

The pictures that play out in our minds are often negative ones that can profoundly affect our heart rate, blood pressure, and stress levels. We picture someone who has angered us, and our blood pressure rises. We imagine an impending argument with the boss, and our body goes into a fight-or-flight response. We see ourselves flubbing a presentation, and butterflies churn in our stomach. Just as negative images can provoke unhealthy reactions, so too can positive images inspire more healthy ones. That's the premise behind guided imagery, a practice that includes visualization.

Fact

In studies, guided imagery has been found to relieve headache pain, improve quality of life for cancer patients, and alleviate stress in postoperative patients. Early research suggests that it can help relieve the pain and fatigue of fibromyalgia.

You can practice guided imagery on your own or with the help of a therapist trained to guide you. Different images work for different people. Some people use images of nature. Others imagine their bodies healing. Others may combine the two. For instance, you might imagine that your pain is the wind, being lifted away into the sky, or water flowing downstream.

If nothing else, guided imagery promotes relaxation and calm and reduces stress, which in turn can help you sleep and lessen your pain. It can also help relax tense muscles. Talk to your health-care practitioner if you are interested in guided imagery. There are also recorded programs that can be very helpful.

Prayer

Nearly half of all Americans turn to prayer when it comes to health, according to a 2004 survey by the National Center for Health Statistics and the National Center for Complementary and Alternative Medicine. In fact, prayer is the most popular form of complementary medicine, ahead of yoga, meditation, tai chi, and qi gong, all of which have a spiritual component.

Essential

Science can't prove it, but some studies suggest that praying for others—also called distant healing—can positively impact those who are sick. And to avoid the placebo effect, or the power of positive thinking, scientists have even demonstrated that prayer can affect the growth of bacteria and seeds.

Praying for good health is nothing new, and for people with a chronic illness like fibromyalgia, it can provide relief. Placing your fate in the hands of a divine power undoubtedly provides comfort for your most difficult moments.

Sometimes, soliciting the prayers of others can enhance your relief. You may solicit prayers through your church or synagogue or from family members. There are even prayer ministries, such as Silent Unity, where associates receive 2 million calls a year from people asking for prayers, most often for health reasons. Callers who report back say they take great comfort in knowing that others are praying with them. But prayer, like meditation, also has a physiologic effect. It slows our heart rate, calms our pulse, and lowers blood pressure. It also relieves stress and anxiety, and can promote a sense of well-being.

Everyone prays in his own unique way and connects to his own higher power. But certain practices can help enhance your prayer experience:

1. Seek out a quiet space alone. The setting should be comfortable and one reserved just for praying.
2. Sit down and slowly get yourself in a relaxed state by focusing on your breath.
3. Begin by expressing gratitude. Acknowledging your blessings can bring you greater joy and help you become more aware of the workings of God or a higher authority.
4. Speak—silently or aloud—words that have meaning to you. That may be a mantra such as "Thy will be done" or a favorite passage from a religious text.
5. Incorporate different types of prayer into your practice. Ask forgiveness, beseech for pain relief, or express adoration. Different forms of prayer will heighten your awareness of a divine power.
6. Consider praying for others. Turning to a higher power on behalf of other people has perks, too. Praying for others, after all, is an act of charity and kindness. "It can bring comfort to you to pray for others," says Harold Koenig, M.D., author of *The Healing Power of Faith*. "It puts your focus on others and off yourself."
7. Make it social. If you prefer the camaraderie of praying with others, consider creating a prayer group or joining one.

Praying with others can strengthen your faith and make the experience more powerful.

8. Commit to a daily practice of five to ten minutes a day and work up to a little longer, if you can.

9. Try to avoid imposing your will on God. Praying for the elimination of your fibromyalgia might make you angry and resentful if it doesn't happen. If, on the other hand, you ask for the strength and willpower to take care of your health, you are much more likely to see results.

Progressive Muscle Relaxation

If your body has been besieged by pain, it may be hard for you to recall what it feels like to have relaxed muscles. All you feel is muscle pain, which has been made worse by your constant clenching and contracting. For some people, progressive muscle relaxation can help you learn the difference between tense and relaxed muscles. Done regularly and correctly, this practice can help you train your muscles to relax.

The technique was developed in 1929 by a psychologist from Chicago named Edward Jacobson, who detailed how to do progressive muscle relaxation. He said it impossible to feel physical pain if the muscles in our body are completely relaxed. Mastering progressive muscle relaxation takes practice, however, especially if you are in pain. Here's how to do it:

1. Locate a quiet place and get into a comfortable position.
2. Close your eyes.
3. Begin by tensing up your toes for five seconds. Then relax them. Notice the different sensation between tensing and relaxing.
4. Progressively move up the body, alternating between tensing, or clenching, and relaxing.
5. Continue all the way up to your head, making sure to also include your shoulders and jaw.

Cognitive-Behavioral Therapy (CBT)

If you're like many people, the way you think is as distressing as any real or imagined event. Cognitive-behavioral therapy (CBT) can help change the way you think and behave in order to minimize stress and anxiety and thereby lessen your symptoms. If your first reaction to a bad flare is to panic, CBT can help you alter those thoughts so that you are not as fretful and so you behave in a way that supports more positive thinking.

CBT combines two kinds of psychotherapy—cognitive therapy and behavior therapy. Cognitive therapy teaches you how certain thought patterns may play a role in worsening your symptoms. For instance, you may be thinking, "Now I'll never be able to play tennis again." These thoughts can trigger anxiety and depression, which only make your pain worse.

 Alert

When you feel pain, try to keep your focus on the present. Avoid thoughts that take you to the future, such as, "How will I possibly get through the meeting tomorrow if I feel like this?" or the past, such as "I knew I shouldn't have gone bike riding yesterday." Shifting your thoughts to other moments in time can often worsen the pain.

CBT helps weaken the link between troublesome situations and your reactions to them. For instance, if you typically react to a flare with rage, your therapist will work with you to change that reaction to one that is more positive. It also teaches you how to calm your mind and body so you can think more clearly and make better decisions. In some ways, CBT is similar to education, coaching, or tutoring.

Other Mind-Body Techniques

Some of the practices we've discussed so far are more formal and may require assistance from a trained practitioner or some research and training by you, the patient. But there are numerous habits and practices that you can incorporate into your daily routine that bolster your mind's power over your body. Francine, for example, has learned to think beyond her pain and to separate her pain from her life.

> Francine said she decided early on that she was going to fight fibromyalgia with all her strength and that she would refuse to let it destroy her life. Bolstered by her faith, family, and friends, Francine learned to separate her pain from what else she was doing, which was always more important than any pain she was feeling. Whether she is busy at her job as a model or talking to people about fibromyalgia, Francine says she tells herself that she is not her pain, but a valuable human being with something to offer the world.

As Francine demonstrates, the way you think can make a world of difference in how you feel. But certain practices can help you reshape your thoughts. Done correctly and regularly, they can relieve your symptoms and improve overall well-being. Although they will not cure you of fibromyalgia, they can help you feel better for the moment. Here are a few of the practices you might consider trying:

- Affirmations—Similar to positive self-talk, affirmations repeated over and over again can help you shift into a more positive frame of mind.
- Deep breathing—Taking deep abdominal breaths over and over makes it almost impossible for your muscles to tense up. So get in the habit of doing that, no matter where you are or what you're doing.
- Relaxation tapes—These tapes, readily available in bookstores and music stores, use music, nature sounds, and soothing voices to help you relax.
- Walking meditation—For those people who have difficulty sitting still, walking while meditating can sometimes be an alternative. While you stroll, focus on your breath, or imagine a place you'd like to be.

Note the Placebo Effect

You've probably heard of the placebo effect. Whether it's your faith in God or your belief in the healing power of biofeedback, some experts think that simply believing—or having faith—that something will work is enough to cause the body to heal. The phenomenon often explains the efficacy of so-called treatments that in reality are nothing but sugar pills or sham surgeries. The idea is that if you believe a therapy will work, then it will, which illustrates yet again the power of positive thought.

In medical research, placebos are sugar pills. One group receives the therapy, the other a placebo. In some studies, however, even a placebo produces the desired effect. For example, one recent study found that patients treated with a placebo for a cough experienced more of an improvement than those who got no treatment.

While the placebo effect may frustrate pharmaceutical companies trying to demonstrate the efficacy of their drugs, you can use the placebo effect to your advantage. Approach the therapies you try with a positive attitude. Have faith that they will help you, even if they don't cure you. Now, that's positive thinking.

CHAPTER 17

Working and Traveling

Holding down a job when you have fibromyalgia isn't easy. You may be in too much pain, or too tired to perform your duties, and the fibro fog can make it hard to concentrate. It's also hard to travel any distance when you have fibromyalgia. In this chapter, we'll take a look at how fibro impacts work and travel and what you can do to make these vital parts of life a little easier.

Working with Fibromyalgia

Doing a job when you have a chronic pain condition can be mentally exhausting and physically taxing. And because fibromyalgia is so variable, it's difficult to know exactly how your condition will influence your function on the job. If your case is mild, it may have no impact on your ability to work. If your job is physically demanding, you may experience some limitations. And if you have a severe case of fibromyalgia, you may have difficulty working at all.

 Fact

If you work alone handling information such as reports, proposals, data, or research, you may be a prime candidate for telecommuting. As of 2004, there were an estimated 44.4 million telecommuters in the United States, according to a survey by the International Telework Association and Council (ITAC).

Certain tasks in particular seem to aggravate fibro symptoms. A study involving 321 fibromyalgia patients found that some tasks were especially difficult, such as computer work or typing, prolonged sitting, prolonged standing and walking, heavy lifting and bending, and repeated moving and lifting. On the other hand, certain activities seemed less likely to worsen fibro symptoms, including walking, variable light sedentary work, teaching, light deskwork, and phone work. It appears that people with fibromyalgia fare best in jobs with tasks that are varied and allow for changes in position.

For some people, simply getting up and going to a job can be exhausting. Take Joy, a security manager who has been battling fibromyalgia for three years.

> Joy knows she would be better off physically if she didn't work. Her job is stressful, and on nights when she doesn't sleep well, Joy feels lousy in the morning. "I know I should sleep longer in the morning to replenish my body but I don't because I really can't," she says. "At work, all I want to do is lie down and sleep for an hour because I'm exhausted." Joy knows she is constantly pushing herself when she should be resting more. And quitting is not an option, because she needs the income and worries she'll get depressed.

Like any person with fibromyalgia, Joy needs to find ways of doing her job that are less stressful. Granted, some things, such as her hours, may be difficult to change. But maybe she can find time to sneak in a ten-minute nap.

To help you resolve difficulties at your job, start by figuring out what exactly is making it hard to work. Everyone is different, and what makes one FMS patient uncomfortable may not necessarily affect another person. Once you identify these challenges, you can work toward identifying solutions. Here are some work-related issues that can often exacerbate the symptoms of fibromyalgia, along with some possible solutions to the problems:

- Repetitive tasks for prolonged periods—Look for opportunities to take short breaks to stretch or relax. Try to alternate the repetitive tasks with other responsibilities in order to break up the repetition.

- One position for extended periods of time—Make a conscious effort to switch positions every few minutes. If you are required to sit, try standing. If you're forced to stand, take time to sit.
- A high-stress work environment—Practice relaxation exercises throughout the day. Deep breaths, guided imagery, and short periods of meditation can help you escape the stress of the moment.
- Computer work that strains your neck, shoulders, and/or back—Enlist an ergonomics specialist to check the positioning of items at your workstation. Make sure everything is at the right height to minimize strain.

If you do a lot of typing on the job, consider trying voice-recognition software. There are a number of computer programs that can automatically transcribe dictation for you. If your job allows it, try one of these programs to cut back on your typing duties. It can save a lot of time, as well as the wear and tear on your hands, arms, and shoulders.

On-the-Job Accommodations

Eventually, some people with fibromyalgia are no longer able to keep doing their jobs. This is often a crushing blow, not only to your household income but also to your ego and sense of self-worth. As a result, you may resist disability for as long as possible. But the reality is that fibromyalgia makes some jobs too difficult to perform.

The good news is, disabled Americans are legally protected under the Americans with Disabilities Act (ADA), a law passed by Congress in 1990. The ADA prohibits employers with fifteen or more employees from discriminating against people with disabilities in making decisions about hiring and employment. In addition to employment, the law means equal opportunity in transportation, public accommodations, state and local government services, and telecommunications. The ADA also has some other rules that can protect you.

If you do need certain accommodations, your employer cannot pay you a lower wage or salary to cover the cost of these accommodations. An employer also can't ask you to pay for these items. If any modification poses undue economic hardship on the employer, the company must offer you the option of providing it yourself or paying for part of it.

An employer cannot ask if you have a disability or about the severity of it. But an employer is allowed to ask if you are able to perform the essential duties of the job.

Before offering you a job, an employer cannot ask you to undergo a medical examination. After a job offer, however, the employer can make that request, provided all employees in that position are required to do the same. Your medical records must remain confidential.

Essential

Occupational therapists can help you figure out ways to make a job adapt to your physical needs and requirements. They can also recommend different types of adaptive equipment to make a job more doable. For more information, check out the American Occupational Therapy Association, Inc., Web site at *www.aota.org*.

Your employer must offer you the same health insurance benefits that are offered to other employees. But an employer is not required to offer you extra benefits to cover your medical condition, and a new insurance carrier may not cover pre-existing conditions.

If it's obvious that you have a disability that will interfere—or already does affect—your ability to perform certain tasks, your employer is entitled to ask you to describe or demonstrate how you would perform the tasks and whether you need any accommodations to help you do them.

At the same time, the ADA does not require employers to make major changes to accommodate your medical condition. Employers do not need to provide accommodations that impose "undue hardship" on business operations, and they are not expected to lower their quality and production standards to accommodate your disability. In addition, employers are not obligated to provide personal use items such as splints or special eyewear for people with disabilities. So although an employer cannot discriminate against you due to a disability, he is allowed to expect the same job performance from you as from a person without a disability.

Who Needs to Know?

To tell or not to tell? That is the question that hovers over many people with fibromyalgia, who wonder whether they should reveal their medical condition to their employers and colleagues. For some people, it may become impossible to keep their condition a secret. Eventually, your difficulties may become apparent. You may also need special accommodations in order to do your job. And if it becomes too much effort for you to keep your fibromyalgia a secret, you may simply want to relieve yourself of the burden of secrecy.

Still, it's important to think it through before deciding to discuss your condition with your employer. What will you gain from your revelation? What might you lose? If you work for a corporation with a strong commitment to helping the disabled, you could benefit from telling your employer. Perhaps you can work out a new schedule or shift from a full-time job to a part-time one. Maybe your employer would allow a job share with another employee.

On the other hand, if you do bring up your condition, you may raise questions about your competence. You may worry that you won't be considered for future promotions, plum positions, and special assignments. You may also encounter subtle forms of discrimination that are almost impossible to prove. With prospective employers, you may be concerned that you'll be dismissed as a job candidate for fear of high medical bills. You may wonder, too, whether your coworkers will treat you differently and resent any special treatment you receive. All of these concerns are factors you should consider before deciding whether to reveal your illness.

 Alert

Avoid overworking yourself just to prove that you can do the job as well as the next person. You may just cause a flare-up. The fact is that the next person may not have fibromyalgia or any other chronic condition. Instead, focus on accepting your limitations and maximizing your effectiveness within them.

For those with significant fibromyalgia, hiding the condition can become too difficult. You may wonder whether you really want to work in such an environment. If not, you may choose to be up front from the beginning. If your honesty keeps you from getting hired at all, it may be just as well.

If you do decide to tell your employer you have fibromyalgia, describe your condition in simple terms and explain how it might affect your work. Many people are still ignorant of fibromyalgia, and you may be educating your boss on the subject. Explain that you are not looking for sympathy, but rather for solutions. It's a good idea to research the kinds of changes you are looking for beforehand.

Working Differently, Working Better

If you are having trouble doing your job, consider speaking with a vocational rehabilitation counselor or social worker. These professionals can help assess your marketable skills and assist in your decision about whether to stay with your current job, find a new job, or train for a new and different profession. In some cases, having fibromyalgia might simply mean doing your job a little differently than you used to. Simply tweaking the way you work can sometimes make all the difference. Here are some tips:

- Pace your workload. Alternate between light tasks and heavy ones.
- Create an efficient workspace. Place things you use frequently within easy reach.
- Conserve energy. Reserve the harder or heavier jobs for the times of day when you feel most energetic.
- Take regular breaks, even when you feel okay. Gentle stretching, relaxation exercises, and short rests can help rejuvenate you.
- Develop working relationships. Trade off tasks that are difficult for you with a coworker.
- Resist the urge to compare yourself with colleagues. Remember, they do not have fibromyalgia.
- If necessary, consider working part-time or from home.
- Be honest with yourself about your ability to do your job. Remember, your health must be a priority.

Before doing anything drastic, like quitting or filing for disability, try and make your job situation more accommodating to your needs. If you're having a major flare, most states have provisions for short-term disability that will allow you to focus on getting yourself better and getting back to full functionality. With some jobs, it may be difficult to make adjustments. Consider the case of Ellen, a preschool teacher in an urban district.

Ellen is the only teacher in a classroom with eighteen four-year olds. So when she isn't feeling well, she does her best to stay off her feet. She also limits the amount of gross motor activities she does with the kids. On days when she's scheduled a visit to the nearby museum, she will cancel the trip and instead take the kids to the playground, where she doesn't have to do so much walking.

For many people, the idea of not working or applying for disability is an absolute last resort. Instead, you might want to consider other ways of working and look for a different job.

If you think you'd like to consider a new career or a different type of job, think about the types of activities that interest you. Then try to envision a dream job. Where would your office be? What kinds of hours would you work? Who would you work with? Talk to career counselors or vocational experts about the types of jobs you might qualify for. Consider getting additional training if necessary. This might be the opportunity for you to create a more ideal work situation.

If You Become Disabled

Estimates suggest that approximately 25 percent of all people with fibromyalgia are receiving disability payments. But applying for disability benefits can be a long, painstaking process that requires patience and perseverance.

 Fact

To help more people with disabilities find work and get vocational services, the Social Security Administration offers the voluntary Ticket to Work Program for people receiving Social Security benefits. Recipients take the ticket to any participating employment network or state vocational rehabilitation office. For more information, check out *www.yourtickettowork.com* or call 1-866-YOURTICKET.

People who become disabled may be eligible for benefits from various agencies. Some of these forms of assistance are temporary and provide short-term help until you find another source of assistance. If you are laid off from your job, for instance, you may collect unemployment. If your fibromyalgia was triggered by a work-related injury—though this may be tough to prove—you may be eligible for worker's compensation. If your family qualifies, you may be eligible for a program called temporary assistance for needy families. But if you are going to be disabled for a year or longer, you may qualify for Social Security Administration (SSA) disability benefits.

Applying for Social Security Disability

The SSA offers two types of assistance to people who are disabled. Social Security Disability Insurance provides benefits to workers under age sixty-five who can no longer work or who have lost income as the result of disability. To qualify, you must have worked for a certain amount of time before applying. The amount you receive will depend on your previous salary. Supplemental Security Income is a program based on needs for people who are disabled and who have limited income. People who receive SSI need not have worked to receive these benefits.

The SSA considers a person disabled if she is unable to do any kind of work for which she is suited. The disability should also be expected to last at least a year or to result in death.

Applying for disability will require the support and assistance of your primary care doctor, who should advise you of your option to file for SSA disability when it becomes apparent that you won't be able to work for the next year. In addition, you will need a specialist in fibro. That person is usually a rheumatologist, though a neurologist or pain management specialist may be considered acceptable, too. You also need an attorney who has significant experience getting benefits for fibromyalgia patients. Given that doctors can't prove that you don't have fibro, the SSA is very reluctant to blithely hand out benefits. An experienced attorney can help you meet all their expectations and minimize the risk of denial.

On your initial application, you'll need to describe the nature of your condition, provide the name of your health-care provider, and give a description of your work background and history. The SSA will then delve further into your claim. The agency will most likely contact your health-care providers for information about your condition. A physician who is skilled at keeping good records can be of great assistance when it comes to securing disability benefits. The SSA will also try to determine your capacity for lifting, walking, standing, and sitting. In addition, you will undergo a physical exam by a physician hired by the SSA.

Question

Do I actually have to be disabled a year to qualify for benefits?
No. According to the SSA, you should apply for benefits as soon as you can. If you are approved, your payments will begin after a five-month waiting period that starts with the month Social Security decides your disability began.

Dealing with Rejection

It often takes six to eight months before you get a response, and the odds are high that your initial claim will be denied. In fact, only about a third of all applications are approved at this initial stage, and almost all fibro applicants are initially rejected. A claim may be denied for myriad reasons. For instance, the SSA may think that you can still perform a different type of job, even if it's the kind of work you have been doing. If your initial claim is denied, you will want to appeal to have your case reconsidered, a process called a request for reconsideration. But it must be done within sixty days of the mailing date of your rejection.

At this point, you may consider hiring an attorney to help with the filing process. The attorneys are generally paid 25 percent of back benefits—monies you would have received if you'd started receiving benefits at the time when you first declared you were unable to work. To find a lawyer, ask your physician for a recommendation or contact the local or state bar association. Approximately 13 percent of cases are awarded disability at this second stage. If your claim is denied a second time, you may request a hearing. Again, the request must be made with sixty days of the mailing date of the appeal rejection. The hearing is usually held before an administrative law judge. During the hearing, you and your doctor may be called upon to testify. At this stage, approximately 68 percent of the cases are approved.

If the judge still determines that you are not disabled, you may take an appeal to the Appeals Council, again within sixty days of the judge's ruling. In most cases, the council's decision typically agrees with the judge's. If you choose, you may file an appeal in U.S. District Court, which may ask for a new hearing.

There's no doubt that the process of getting Social Security benefits can be lengthy and exhausting. But considering that you may be eligible for as much as $1,000 a month, the process is well worth the trouble. And once you're approved for Social Security payments, you will become eligible for Medicare, the government-sponsored health insurance program. You will receive Medicare benefits after you've gotten disability benefits for twenty-four months. For more information on Social Security, check out the Web site at *www.ssa.gov*.

Essential

To help health-care professionals better understand disabling medical conditions, the Social Security Administration publishes a book called *Disability Evaluation Under Social Security*, also known as the *Blue Book*. When ruling on a case, the SSA relies in part on this 187-page document. As of now, fibromyalgia is not specifically included on the list. To download a copy, go to *www.ssa.gov/disability/ professionals/bluebook*.

Don't let the daunting nature of applying for benefits deter you. Keep in mind that you did not choose to become disabled and that you are merely trying to attain benefits that are rightfully yours. At the same time, be level headed. Keep good records, and stay cool and calm during any interviews.

Traveling with Fibro

The idea of jet-setting anywhere might be the last thing on your mind. But imagine lounging poolside at a Hawaiian resort, shopping and sightseeing in a historic town, or simply visiting special friends. When you're sick, a vacation getaway can be just what you need to alleviate your stress.

Having fibromyalgia doesn't mean you have to stop traveling. It simply means you'll need to plan carefully so you'll remember your medications and any other special devices you use. It means strategizing, so that you don't overdo it and tire yourself out. It might also mean adjusting your vacation plans a bit so that you don't sap your energy. Belinda, for instance, began making plans for her trip months in advance, knowing she wanted to go hiking.

> To celebrate their twenty-fifth wedding anniversary, Belinda and her husband chose to go to Hawaii. She knew she wanted to go hiking. To prepare her body, Belinda began doing some gentle weight training with a skilled trainer, who knew about fibromyalgia. But she also knew that she'd have to conserve her energy if she wanted to survive the hike. She resisted the urge to stop in California and spent the first two days in Hawaii recovering from the flight. And when she got home, she made sure to schedule nothing the first few days, except a hot stone massage.

As Belinda demonstrates, you can enjoy traveling, so long as you plan ahead. Plotting for a successful trip can make all the difference in how you feel before, during, and after your travels.

Travel by Plane or Train

Traveling is easier than ever in this day and age. But for someone with fibromyalgia, it may seem daunting. If you're planning to fly or take a train, make reservations early. Consider requesting your seat assignment when you book the flight. Ask for seating that provides more legroom, such as the first seat or one in an exit row. If possible, avoid peak times of the day, like the morning or late afternoon, when airports and train stations are busiest.

Also, try to book a nonstop direct flight to avoid the inconvenience of transferring to another plane in an unfamiliar airport. If you have no choice, find out how long it will take you to get to your connecting flight. Then request additional time between your flights when booking your ticket or make arrangements to get there by way of an electric cart.

When traveling, always dress comfortably, especially when it comes to footwear. Long lines are common at airports. If possible, arrange to preboard the plane or train. Most airlines will allow passengers with disabilities to board in advance. Ask your doctor for a letter if you think you'll need to convince airport personnel of your disability. And don't hesitate to ask for help. Some airports provide electric carts or trams that will take you to the gate.

 Alert

Steer clear of water in airplane bathrooms. Studies by the Environmental Protection Agency have found that the water from the tap of an aircraft bathroom is contaminated with disease-causing organisms. So carry a bottle of drinking water with you in your carry-on luggage. After using the toilet, wash with soap and water, and then apply an antibacterial gel.

On the flight or train, always keep medications and other personal items with you in the event there is a delay or your luggage is lost. Also, be sure to bring along some food and a bottle of water, especially if you need it to take your medications. That way you're not stuck relying on the airplane attendants to serve you when you need to take your drugs. You're also not forced to navigate a bumpy train to get in line at the cafeteria car.

No matter how you travel, make time to get up and walk around. Do some simple range-of-motion exercises if you can. Booking an aisle seat can make this much easier.

Travel by Car

If you do wind up driving to your destination, be sure to build in time for rest stops. Don't sit in a car for more than thirty to sixty minutes at a time, depending on the severity of your condition. Pull over at rest areas, picnic parks, or gas stations, and walk around.

If you do drive, make sure to adapt your vehicle to maximize your comfort. Install special wide-angle side and rear-view mirrors to increase your field of view without having to twist and turn around in the driver's seat. Use a cushioned seat belt for more shoulder comfort. Cover your steering wheel in sheepskin so you can use a looser grip. If you're renting a vehicle and can afford it, choose a van, so that you can get up and move around periodically.

To provide added support and pain relief, use pillows and cushions. Cervical collars can help lessen neck pain, while a lumbar pillow can provide lower back support. You can also use cushions for sore hips and backs.

Strategies for Any Trip

Whenever you travel, research your destinations, and zero in on the activities you want to do. Call the hotels ahead of time and find out the kinds of amenities they have. For instance, if you enjoy water exercises, you might want to find out if they have a pool or whirlpool. You might also want to find out whether they have a blow dryer, laundry facilities, or other amenities, so you don't need to pack anything extra.

Always travel as lightly as possible. Plan to do laundry on your trip and to purchase some items at your destination so you can minimize your packing. Lightweight luggage on wheels is a must, as it is easier to transport in busy hotels and airports.

Before you take off, be sure to let your traveling companions or hosts know that you need time to rest and relax upon your arrival and throughout your trip. Be honest about how much activity you can really handle. Always take time to rest. The last thing you want is a fibro flare-up to ruin your excursion.

CHAPTER 18

Fibromyalgia and Your Relationships

A major chronic illness can reshape the way others perceive you as well as the way you relate to them. But don't underestimate the impact of these relationships on your life. A strong, solid support network can make a world of difference in how you fare with fibromyalgia. On the other hand, the lack of support can be detrimental to your health. In this chapter, we look at how fibro can affect your most critical relationships.

New Ways of Coping

Before you became ill, you may have invested a lot of time and energy in your relationships. The energy you devoted to people you love probably came very easily to you. When you have a chronic illness like fibromyalgia, your priorities must naturally shift. Now that you have fibromyalgia, taking care of yourself has to come first. Think of the announcement you hear each time you board an airplane, when the flight attendants ask that you put the oxygen mask on yourself before tending to your children. The same philosophy applies with fibromyalgia. Only by caring for yourself first are you able to continue nurturing the relationships in your life.

For some people, this shift is difficult. You may be accustomed to thinking of others first. What will little Johnny do if he can't make it to soccer practice? How will the committee function if you're not there to take notes? How will your spouse prepare a meal if you can't make dinner? At the very least, you probably gave as much as you took and often traded off tasks with friends and loved ones, so that everyone could get things done.

But having FMS requires that you put yourself first and foremost; your health must take center stage over anything else you do. Trying to convince loved ones, friends, colleagues, and employers of this new shift can be difficult, however, especially when you don't appear to be sick. Some may never understand and will simply drift away. Others may get hostile, taking your absence as a sign that you no longer care about them. Still others may hear you out but not really grasp the severity of your condition. But the ones who truly care will stand by you and help you make these adjustments.

L. Essential

Major change—like moving or having kids—always tests the strength of existing relationships. And sometimes some friendships do fall by the wayside. Keep in mind that having fibromyalgia can open up other doors and introduce new people into your life—if you let them in.

When you have a chronic disease, it's easy to feel lonely. Friends may have a difficult time understanding the true extent of your pain and fatigue. Your children may not comprehend the difficulties you face. Your spouse may be overwhelmed, even terrified by the prospect of spending his life with someone battling a strange medical condition.

That's why it's so important to find or create the support you need. Whether it's an existing relationship with a spouse or a close friend, or a new one with a support group, a strong network of social support is important to your health. It may buffer you from the pain of a flare-up, buoy you on days when your spirits are down, and help redirect your attention and energies elsewhere. A solid support network offers a palliative that no pharmaceutical can ever deliver.

Fibro and Your Marriage

Any marriage or intimate relationship has its shares of normal ups and downs. But being diagnosed with a condition like fibromyalgia creates dramatic additional challenges and strains. When you have fibromyalgia, your spouse has to accept you as a somewhat different person, someone whose energy may be limited and whose skills may be reduced. For some people, this transition can be difficult. Your spouse may mistake your fatigue for a lack of interest in what's going on in his life and your pain as an excuse for getting out of chores. It may be hard for him to realize and accept just how sick you are, especially if you have no outward symptoms.

Enduring a medical condition like fibromyalgia tests a couple's resilience. If you're lucky, your partner will make an effort to understand what you are experiencing and ask how he or she can help. Some people, like Gina, are blessed with a spouse who does all he can to help.

Although few of her extended family members understood fibromyalgia, Gina's husband Richard always did. "My husband is a godsend," says Gina, who has had fibro for more than twenty years. "He looks in my eyes and knows exactly what's going on. Even when I'm trying to tell him that I'm okay, he can always tell when I'm not." During her worst battles with fibro, Richard worked a full-time job, then came home and made dinner. It was at his urging that Gina stopped working for a while.

Not everyone has a spouse like Richard. But you can help build your spouse's empathy by educating him about the disease and keeping lines of communication wide open. It can also help to bring your partner to doctor's appointments. Not only will your partner develop a better understanding of your illness, but he may be better equipped to help you make decisions about it if he's involved in your medical care.

Don't forget that your partner is coming to terms with fibromyalgia as well. He may not be able to understand exactly how you feel and may be uncertain of how to approach you. Should he offer help? Give you advice? Should he talk about your condition at all or act as if nothing was any different? That's why you need to set the tone of your relationship early on. After all, you're the one confronting the pain, fatigue, and limitations of fibromyalgia. Only you can tell your partner what you want and need from him.

Whether it's asking your partner to handle the housecleaning on your bad days or expressing your concerns over your ability to keep working, talking to your partner is more critical now than ever. If you don't want him to offer you advice, tell him so. If you'd rather he not discuss it with his friends, let him know that. Don't expect that love alone will produce the kind of understanding you need. You have to speak up and make yourself heard.

At the same time, be attentive to your spouse, too. Make sure your partner is taking care of himself. Remind him to exercise, eat well, and pursue activities that he enjoys on his own. Don't expect him to devote every waking moment to tending to your needs. And make sure you express appreciation for your partner's support. A simple thank you can sometimes go a long way.

Essential

No one wants to help a constant whiner who isn't doing her best to take care of her health. So make sure you give it your all when it comes to making doctor appointments, exercising, and taking your medications. By showing others that you're making a sincere effort to get well, you'll win their support.

It's also important to realize that there will be times when your partner's compassion is tapped out. Any person can give only so much support, and your needs may overwhelm his capacity. Unfortunately, it's easy to interpret this as abandonment, prompting a response from you that can lead to a major argument. Instead, agree beforehand to a term he can use when he's used up, such as, "Honey, I'd love to be here for you now, but my batteries are drained. Can you call a friend?" By agreeing beforehand, you'll understand what's going on with him and accept it much more easily.

Having Sex

Cozying up to your spouse or partner may be the last thing on your mind when you're battling fibromyalgia. Painful muscles, headaches (real ones!), fatigue, and other symptoms can make it hard to muster the energy for sex. Add to that the effects of medications and the stress of being ill, and you have a recipe for low sex drive.

 Alert

Certain medications can zap your libido and make it difficult for you to enjoy sex. The antidepressant Prozac, for example, can interfere with orgasms and dampen desire. If you suspect a medication may be affecting your sex drive, talk to your doctor about switching to another drug.

It's not at all unusual for couples dealing with fibromyalgia to have problems in their sex life. Having fibromyalgia can affect self-esteem and cause depression, which can make it difficult to even think about having sex. Even if the desire is there, it can be difficult if your muscles hurt or if you suffer from vulvodynia. In some cases, sex can mean heightened mental alertness and lack of sleep. In other people, sex can cause more pain.

But the absence of sex in an intimate relationship can be a threat to that relationship. To sustain an active sex life, keep your lines of communication open. Let your partner know how fibromyalgia has affected your desire and ability to have sex. Discuss ways that you do enjoy being touched and other ways of being intimate that may not involve intercourse. Explore different positions for having sex that may be less painful. Do not have sex when you're in the throes of pain, since that may only build resentment and disrupt the relationship.

If necessary, try planning for sex. Granted, it may not be as exciting or spontaneous. But planning can make it happen. On the days that you do have sex, conserve your energy during the day so that you will be less fatigued at night. Make time for a warm bath so that you can reduce pain and stiffness.

Couples can also practice a technique called sensate focusing, a type of erotic intimacy that involves different types of touch while delaying touch of the erogenous zones. It can be very helpful to do gentle caresses, or touching with a soft object like a cotton ball, feather, or warm water. Sensate focusing helps get you back into your body in a pleasant, desirable way and can open the door to greater sexual intimacy.

Remember, keeping the intimacy alive in a relationship doesn't have to be simply about sex. The key is to spend time doing things together that forge intimacy, like snuggling on a couch or holding hands while taking a walk. However, if you do have the energy and desire for sex, then by all means, indulge. Orgasms release feel-good endorphins that can help temporarily distract you from your pain.

Communication: The Key

Not everyone has an easy time expressing feelings. Some people may keep difficult emotions bottled up. Others may have a hard time asking others for help. Still others may know what they want to say but have a hard time putting it into a clear message. Stella, for example, is still embarrassed to admit when fibro interferes with her plans.

> Stella has suffered from fibromyalgia for about fifteen years. Six years ago, she was diagnosed with rheumatoid arthritis, too. Though her family is well aware of her limitations, she still isn't comfortable discussing it with some of her friends. Not long ago, she and her husband cancelled their ballroom dance lessons because her legs and feet hurt. When her friend called to ask where they were, Stella said she was having problems with her health. "But I felt funny admitting it," Stella says. "It felt like a cop-out." She only recently began accepting help for the annual Thanksgiving dinner, which she used to prepare by herself. Now everyone brings a dish, Stella says.

As Stella finally learned, the only way to make your wishes heard is to speak up. If friends want you to join them on an outing you really have no energy for, you need to say so. If your boss expects you to stay late, and you're too tired, you'll need to let him know and work out an alternative. When your kids want you to take them to the mall, and you can't muster the strength, you have to tell them that you simply can't do it. Don't expect others to be mind readers.

Some people have a difficult time asking for help. But when you have a disease like fibromyalgia, you will need help from others, especially loved ones. Get in the habit of asking directly for what you want, without making someone feel guilty, playing the martyr, or antagonizing the recipient of your message. The key is to describe exactly what you need and what you expect from the other person. And to ensure you get the help you want, toss in some appreciation for the other person's efforts. A little charm goes a long way.

Fibromyalgia and Children

It's never easy when chronic illness affects a child. Although the focus of this book is on adults with fibromyalgia, the condition can also affect children, be it directly or when a parent has it. In either case, fibromyalgia can cause tremendous stress for a young child.

Fact

According to the Arthritis Foundation, approximately 10,000 children are diagnosed with fibromyalgia each year, most of them adolescents. Although the symptoms are similar, children generally have fewer tender points. Among adults who have fibromyalgia, most can remember early symptoms that began in their childhood.

Children who have fibromyalgia have many of the same symptoms that adults do—pain, fatigue, and difficulties concentrating. They may experience trouble sleeping and have restless legs syndrome. They may become depressed and anxious about being sick. They may also experience numbness, dizziness, and tingling.

As the parent of a child with fibromyalgia, you are your child's advocate. It is up to you to meet with doctors and health-care professionals to discuss your child's care and treatment. It is also up to you to speak with teachers and other adults about the impact of fibro on your child's ability to function and perform.

If your child has fibromyalgia, teach her how to cope by eating well, resting when necessary, and keeping stress at bay. Don't shield her from the reality of her condition, but do use simple words to explain it so she understands.

When Mom or Dad Has Fibro

Parenting has never been an easy job. But trying to parent when you have fibromyalgia can become extremely difficult, especially during bad flare-ups. You may not be able to do as much as you could before you got sick. And the fluctuating nature of the disease makes it hard to give your children the structure and consistency they need.

Essential

Children may be frightened to learn that a parent is sick. Some may worry that you will die. But don't be afraid to tell them about fibromyalgia. Let them know that you will have good days and bad days, that you won't die from it, and that you will still be available to them. Give them opportunities to discuss their fears and concerns, too.

If your children are old enough, tell them you have fibromyalgia in terms they can understand. Explain what the disease does and how it makes you hurt and tired. Let them know that you will have days when the pain is worse or better and that there may be activities you can no longer do. Encourage them to discuss how they feel about your illness so they have a place to vent frustrations.

Don't be hesitant to ask your children for help, if they're old enough to perform chores. Most children welcome the ability to contribute when given the chance. The additional responsibilities will even help foster their sense of responsibility.

Once your kids are older and start forming friendships, don't hesitate to enlist the help of other parents if you're having difficulty getting your kids to parties and activities. In return, offer to help out in other ways on days when you're feeling good. Again, the key is to speak up and communicate your needs. Don't sit back and expect that people will offer, even if they know you have fibromyalgia. Only you know the pain and difficulties you're experiencing.

Whatever you do, eliminate the guilt that comes with not being able to be the parent you might have planned to be. Children are skilled at sensing parental guilt and may use it to manipulate you. Keep in mind that no one, not even a healthy person, is the perfect parent. If you look around closely at other families, you'll see that parenting poses challenges for everyone. Yours just happens to be fibromyalgia.

Maintaining Friendships

In the midst of severe pain and fatigue, you may want little to do with the outside world, preferring instead to hide inside your house. While a little rest can be good for you, it can be easy to overdo it. Staying isolated on a regular basis isn't good for your health. That's why you need friendships that nourish your spirit.

But when you have fibromyalgia—or any chronic condition, for that matter—you need to be more selective about the friends you see. Friends that sabotage your feelings and make light of your pain will only cause stress, which is certainly something you don't need. You need to surround yourself with friends who are willing to listen to your concerns and feelings, and who will give you encouragement and hope when you need it. You need friends who will offer advice when you need it, but who will stay silent when you don't.

At the same time, steer clear of people who minimize your condition or who make you feel you must put on a cheerful front, no matter how bad you really feel. Avoid people who are uncomfortable discussing your condition or who give you too much pity. These people are more likely to make you feel bad about yourself.

The goal is to be selective about how you spend your social time, especially since it's now become more limited and precious. Devote your time and energy to being with people who offer you the support and encouragement you need, people whose very presence brings you true joy. Avoid those who sap your energy and who make you feel bad. Cecilia says she had to let several of her friends go when they had no tolerance for her suffering.

> Ever since she learned she had fibromyalgia, Cecilia has figured out that she needs positive energy in her life to make her feel good. For Cecilia, that has meant saying goodbye to some former friends who didn't understand what she was going through with fibromyalgia and accused her of complaining all the time. But Cecilia has found new friendships through a yoga class she takes, where everyone knows she has fibromyalgia and accepts her.

Fibro Support Groups

Friends and family may be wonderfully supportive as you wrestle with the ups and downs of fibromyalgia. But sometimes, getting together with other people experiencing fibromyalgia lets you know that you aren't suffering alone. Support groups are also a wonderful place to pick up practical advice and strategies for coping. The combined experience of a group can be invaluable in helping you find an understanding doctor, physical therapist, or counselor. Many people wind up making lasting friendships through these groups as members open up about their condition.

Some of the more formal groups may invite guest speakers to come and discuss an aspect of fibromyalgia. Some groups may also involve family members and friends, which is an opportunity for you to educate someone. Many groups use the meetings as a chance to socialize as well, and members bring refreshments to the gatherings.

Unfortunately, some of these get-togethers can become focused on complaining. One member gripes about the way a doctor treated her, and the next thing you know, the entire discussion is focused on lambasting the medical profession. Sometimes it's healthy to vent a little if something has upset you. But if a group is in the habit of complaining, then maybe you should consider a different group. Support groups should support you, not bring you down. Those that are overly negative and hostile will only dredge up your own unhappiness, and that's the last thing you need.

So where do you find a support group? Start by asking your doctor if he knows of one. Some medical practices may even assemble a support group so patients have a forum for sharing ideas. You can also find support groups through a local hospital or national organizations such as the Arthritis Foundation and the National Fibromyalgia Association. These groups can be found on the Web at *www.arthritis.org* and *www.fmaware.org*.

A good support group usually has a facilitator, someone who knows how to redirect the meeting if people get off topic or drone on about something irrelevant. The leader should also give everyone the opportunity to speak and make new members feel welcome. She should also be well versed in fibromyalgia and make sure that accurate information is disseminated.

Not everyone, however, can get to a support group. If you're one of those people, there is support available on the Internet. Many Web sites now host chat rooms and message boards where you can communicate with others about having fibromyalgia. For a listing of medical forums that offer chat rooms, check out *http://members.aol .com/fibrocloud/chat.htm*. The site links to several Web sites that host chat rooms and forums, including iVillage, Oprah, and WebMD.

Creating a Support Network

In her book *Fibromyalgia and Chronic Myofascial Pain*, Devin Starlanyl advises readers to create a group of at least five supporters, so that no one person is called upon to do too much or called upon all the time. And different supporters can perform different roles. One might prepare meals for you. Another might provide a listening ear. Still another might offer medical advice and strategies for coping. All supporters, she says, should meet the following criteria for you:

- You enjoy being with them.
- You choose to be with them when you want to relax and have a good time.
- You turn to them when you need to talk to someone.
- You turn to them for help in making decisions.
- You depend on them for help with tasks in daily living that have become too difficult.

Whether these people are family members, friends, neighbors, or work colleagues, they should all be educated about fibromyalgia and its impact on your life. Tell them that there are times when your pain is severe and the fatigue is overwhelming. Explain that you may not always be able to do all the fun things that they'd like you to do. Tell them that there may be times when you'd prefer to be home lying on the couch than out and about.

Alert

Just because you have the ear and support of a good friend doesn't mean you should take advantage of that relationship. Be vigilant about courtesy and good manners. Don't call too late or expect that person to be available to you at all times. Respect her wish for time with her family. Don't drop in unannounced. She needs to know that her needs are as important to you as yours are to her.

At the same time, don't forget to hold up your end of the relationship. Although relationships must be fifty-fifty, your half of the bargain will need to be made up of activities your fibromyalgia allows you to do. So offer a listening ear or a helping hand whenever you can. And most important, express your gratitude. A simple thank you will let your supporters know that you appreciate them.

CHAPTER 19

Positive Coping

As you already know, it isn't easy living with fibromyalgia. The condition is a constant companion, one that requires vigilant attention and appropriate self-care. But with the right attitude, strategies, and medical care, you can assume some semblance of control over your condition. In this chapter, we'll review some of the most important strategies for living with fibromyalgia.

Take Responsibility

Even before you got sick, you knew that your health was your responsibility. After all, who else will ensure that you exercise, eat right, and go to the doctor for your regular appointments? Now that you have fibromyalgia, those stay-healthy efforts have intensified. On top of exercising regularly, eating well, and going to the doctor's, you may now attend a support group. You may be practicing tai chi to ease your pain and meditating to keep stress at bay. You may even be taking small naps every afternoon to make sure you conserve your energy.

One of the most important things you can do is to take responsibility for your condition. Taking responsibility means assuming control of your health and well-being to the best of your ability. It means doing everything within your power to ensure that you are as healthy as you can be. It means making a commitment to yourself to do what you can to avoid flare-ups and manage your symptoms. For your efforts, you will be rewarded with a greater sense of control and competence over your condition.

Of course, there will be times when this is difficult to do. Severe bouts of fatigue and pain can sabotage your best intentions, and you may become frustrated and annoyed by your seeming inability to positively impact your health. Getting through these difficult periods will test your fortitude, but they are unfortunately a part of the illness. The ability to endure and persevere during these times is also an essential part of staying well. So what does it mean to take responsibility for your health as you learn to live with fibromyalgia? Here is a summary of what you need to do.

Get Educated

As someone living with fibromyalgia, you should learn as much as you can about your condition. The fact you're reading this book and have gotten this far is a great indication of your commitment to becoming more knowledgeable about fibromyalgia. At the same time, you should also continue to stay on top of current research and trends.

Knowing about fibromyalgia will help you recognize the signs and symptoms of fibro and to also distinguish those that are not a result of FMS. It will enable you to speak intelligently about fibromyalgia with family members, health-care professionals, and employers. It will help you ask the right questions when it comes to getting the best care.

Essential

A good place to learn about fibromyalgia is on the Internet, which is rich with health information. But be wary of sites selling particular products or those that promise miracle cures for fibro. Try to stick with the Web sites of well-regarded fibro organizations like the National Fibromyalgia Association, at *www.fmaware.org*.

Most importantly, your knowledge about fibromyalgia will help you take care of yourself. You'll know which drugs to avoid, which exercises to do with caution, and when to call the doctor about a change in your condition. Making the effort to learn about FMS will also benefit those around you, who will come to develop a better understanding of your needs.

Join Your Medical Team

In Chapter 4, we discussed the importance of assembling a good medical team. Now that you have put together a solid team, you need to work with them to make sure you get the appropriate care you need. That means making regular appointments, staying alert to your symptoms, taking your medications as prescribed, and keeping good records of your doctor visits, symptoms, and treatments.

Effective fibromyalgia treatment depends in large part on what you tell your doctor. That's why it's so important for you to keep track of what is happening with your health. So before any visit with a physician, jot down any symptoms, side effects, or concerns. Write down questions about treatments, supplements, or therapies you may hear about. Make a list of all treatments that you have tried, what the dosages were, and why you're no longer on them. Keep a complete list of the medications and supplements you're currently taking, too. Bring your notes to the doctor so you remember everything that needs to be discussed.

Finally, follow your doctor's advice and recommendations. It's frustrating for a physician to offer advice and then find that the patient has chosen to ignore it. If you don't want to do something a doctor recommends, say so, and try to find alternatives. But be open minded. Remember: No treatment can possibly help you if you don't try it. The idea is to work alongside your medical team to come up with ways of coping with your symptoms.

Exercise Regularly

If there's one therapy that everyone agrees can help, it's exercise. Regular physical activity can boost your energy, improve your sleep, enhance your function, and make you less stiff. It can also relieve stress and anxiety. Overall, it can improve your quality of life.

You may wonder how you can possibly exercise when you feel as if you're going to collapse just walking to the mailbox? It's frustrating when your body isn't able to perform the way it once did. But exercise for people with fibromyalgia does not mean what you might think it does. We're not advising that you train for a marathon, bike fifteen miles, or swim fifty laps, even if you could do that in the past. In reality, exercise for people with fibromyalgia might mean gentle stretching, a short walk, or water aerobics in a warm pool.

Alert

When you start to exercise, always begin slowly. If you can't carry on a normal conversation while you're exercising, chances are that you're overdoing it. Slow down, and resume at a gentler pace. Remember to always build up gradually when doing any exercise.

The key is to find out what exercises work for you and to commit to doing them on a regular basis. That might involve working with a physical therapist or a trainer who specializes in fibromyalgia to pin down the exact workout for you. It might also involve a great deal of trial and error before you find the activity that works best. Whatever you do, don't give up. Exercise is important on many levels. With patience and perseverance, you can find an activity that will work to your advantage.

Keep Positive

It isn't easy to remain upbeat and positive in the face of overwhelming pain and fatigue. In fact, it's much easier to become discouraged, depressed, and frustrated. But when it comes to living with fibromyalgia, a positive attitude goes a long way toward getting you well and keeping you there. Telling yourself that you will be okay is much more hopeful and promising than saying, "I'll never get better." But getting yourself to think positively when life looks bleak is difficult and takes practice. To stay positive, you have to keep stress in check, obliterate toxic thoughts that drag your emotions down, and learn to feel good about yourself.

Manage Stress

Nothing sabotages a positive outlook faster than stress, especially when there's too much of it. And let's face it, having a chronic condition like fibromyalgia is certain to cause stress in even the calmest people. You've got too much to do—and no energy to do it. You can't remember anything. To top it off, you're hurting all over. And in addition to your health problems, you've got the kids, the job, and the house. It feels as if the world is crashing in on you, and there's nothing you can do.

Too much stress is hurtful, especially for people who have fibromyalgia. Stress can worsen your pain and fatigue and make it hard to sleep. It can also worsen your fibro fog. In addition, it can make you neglectful of healthy habits so that you wind up eating poorly, forgetting to take medications, and abandoning your exercise regimen.

Beating stress isn't easy, but it can be done. Start by making a commitment to rein in your stress. Keep in mind that as someone with fibromyalgia, for you it is critical to tame your stress. Then make the effort to get it under control with these strategies:

- Set priorities. Focus on what matters most—like your health and your family—and learn to let everything else go.
- Change the way you perceive stressful events. A traffic jam isn't a headache. It's a chance to listen to your favorite music.
- Make time for relaxation. You book everything else in your calendar, so why not make relaxation a part of your day, too?
- Practice positive self-talk. Negative statements can perpetuate your stress. Try talking to yourself with positive comments.

- Maintain a sense of humor. Watch a funny sitcom, or spend time with a friend who makes you laugh.
- Practice deep breathing. Regular deep breathing can lower your stress level and improve your mood.
- Be realistic. Creating unrealistic standards and goals will set you up for disappointment and—you got it—more stress.
- Learn to say no. Don't overcommit yourself. This will come easier once your priorities are in place.

Conquer Difficult Thoughts and Emotions

Everyone knows the emotions that make us feel bad. Anger. Sadness. Frustration. Guilt. All these feelings can make it hard for you to stay positive. But they're also common emotional reactions to having fibromyalgia.

The goal in conquering your difficult emotions isn't to deny them. Instead, you want to channel them so that they don't take over your life. Rather than try to suppress these feelings, try to work through them. Talk them over with a close friend or relative. Write them down in a journal. Acknowledge these emotions, and then move on. If your emotions become overwhelming, seek professional help from a therapist, psychologist, or psychiatrist. In addition, learn to recognize the thoughts that aggravate negative emotions. Always thinking negatively will just drag you into a cesspool of misery. Learning to see when you're getting caught in these traps can help you choose not to fixate on them.

Boost Your Self-Esteem

It's easy to feel badly about yourself when you're sick with fibromyalgia. After all, you may no longer be able to do all the things that you used to do. As a result, you may wonder if you did something to deserve this as you become increasingly frustrated by your illness.

If fibromyalgia has devastated your confidence and self-esteem, it may take a while for you to recover and feel good about yourself. You'll need to uncover or develop new skills and abilities that help mend your confidence. Perhaps you'll realize that you are a truly good friend or an uncommonly good listener. Maybe you'll discover that you're a skilled researcher in your quest for more medical knowledge. Or maybe you'll simply learn that you are a kind person. In any case, you can rebuild your self-esteem as you learn to adjust to having fibromyalgia. Here are some ways to do that:

- Focus on what you can do, not what you can no longer do.
- Explore other interests and hobbies.
- Set realistic goals.
- Do some self-coaching with daily affirmations and positive self-talk.
- Spend time with people who make you feel good about yourself and recognize your inherent worth.

When you develop a chronic illness like fibromyalgia, it's more important than ever to separate who you are from what you do. You are not just a mother/wife/job title. You are not just a doting parent, a good cook, or a skilled worker. You are also a person, a worthwhile and interesting person who just happens to have a chronic illness. The fact you have fibromyalgia should not define who you are; rather, it is just one circumstantial aspect of your character.

Tap Into Your Social Network

Being ill with fibromyalgia can become a lonely venture if you choose to isolate yourself from others. It's true that most people won't be able to imagine the extent of your pain and fatigue. But there's no reason for anyone to endure the rigors of fibromyalgia alone. That's why it's so important to tap into your social supports during this difficult time. Keep in mind, though, that it might be hard for family and friends to offer you their support. Fibromyalgia is not a visible condition, and you may appear perfectly fine to them. The condition also varies from day to day, making it hard for them to understand why you are energetic one day and bedridden the next.

L. Essential

Connecting with other people need not mean a major social outing. A simple phone call or e-mail exchange can help you stay connected during those times when you're in too much pain to get out. If you prefer to see people in person, invite some friends over for coffee. Just don't fret about cleaning.

Just as you need to be educated about fibromyalgia, so too should the people around you. Give them books and articles to read. Bring them along to doctor's appointments and support groups. Help them understand that fibromyalgia remains a medical mystery, one that has no cure but that will remain with you for the rest of your life. And don't forget that your condition will take a toll on your loved ones, too, especially family members who live in the same household. They may be worried, frightened, and sad that you are sick. They may be frustrated by your limitations and afraid of how fibro will affect your future. They may resent doing tasks that once were yours. More than ever, your family will need to come together and provide each other with much-needed support as everyone rallies to help you get well.

Ask for Help

Utilizing your social network means relying a little more on your loved ones, which might include your spouse, your children, or your parents. It might also mean involving friends, neighbors, and colleagues for extra help. You might need your spouse to do more housework, a neighbor to help walk the dog, and a friend to listen while you vent your frustrations. All of these are ways that you can put your social network to work for you.

It's not always easy to ask others for help. But trying to do it all yourself will only jeopardize your health. So when others offer help, take them up on it. Assign them specific jobs like weeding your garden, going grocery shopping, or preparing a meal.

Don't hesitate to put your children to work, too. Even young children can help with emptying wastebaskets, picking up rooms, and folding laundry. Don't expect that they—or anyone else for that matter—will do things the same way you would. Just be grateful that someone is there to help pick up where you left off.

Create Support

Not everyone has loved ones living nearby or even in the same household. If that's your case, you will need to make a special effort to create a support network. Participate in support groups for others living with fibromyalgia. Develop a phone network with other fibro sufferers. Consider hiring some help. Enlist the help of acquaintances for small tasks. If you belong to a church or synagogue, talk to the leader about ways that members might be able to help you.

 Alert

Striving for perfection can be hazardous to your health! The need to be perfect—or at least appear perfect—can cause a host of health problems, including depression, anxiety, and eating disorders. So resist the urge to be perfect or to expect others to meet your standards of perfection. It will only cause unnecessary stress and strain your relationships.

When you do win over the help of others, be kind and supportive in return. On days when you feel less pain, take time to express your gratitude by baking someone a pie, offering to do something for someone else, or sending a thank-you note. In order to receive support, remember that you need to offer support, too.

Aim for Balance

These days, it's not uncommon to read articles about the well-balanced life. It seems that everyone is striving for a perfect blend of activity and rest, solitude and friendship, work and play. In reality, many people are frantically bustling through their days, going from one item on the to-do list to the next, with no real balance at all.

When you have fibromyalgia, living a balanced life becomes much more important. In fact, balance may be critical to your health. But striking the perfect balance takes practice. It also takes time to figure out what works for you. Some people may require more rest, while others are able to withstand more activity. Those who have high-stress jobs may need to devote more time to meditation and relaxation exercises. The idea is to find the best balance for your situation.

To help you attain some sense of balance in your life, figure out how you're spending your time. Are you devoting too much energy to your job? Do you spend too much effort cleaning your house and not enough taking care of your health? Do you make time for yourself on a regular basis, or is all your time devoted to your husband and kids?

Once you start to see where things are out of balance, make an effort to restore some equilibrium to your life. If you work too much, try cutting back your hours. If you put too much emphasis on a clean house, look for ways to cut corners or hire someone to help do the cleaning. If your family occupies the bulk of your life, make sure to squeeze in some time just for you.

Putting It All Together

Getting used to the idea of having fibromyalgia will take some time. It will also take some time for you to conquer stress, learn about your condition, and find the right support systems. But that's okay. Learning to live with a chronic health problem is a process, not something that occurs overnight, in a week, or even in a month. In some cases, it may take years.

By gradually laying the groundwork, though, you can begin to live more amicably with fibromyalgia. No, it is not an easy illness to live with. And until science develops a better understanding of the causes of fibromyalgia and develops better treatments, there will not be easy answers. In the meantime, stay focused on improving your life today.

CHAPTER 20

The Future of Fibro

It's only natural to look to the future in the hopes of a greater understanding of fibromyalgia and the promise of a cure. And right now, the future does indeed look promising—several pharmaceutical companies are exploring new and better treatments for fibro. In this chapter, we'll take a glimpse of what's to come as scientists continue learning about this baffling illness.

Treatments on the Horizon

Scientists in research laboratories around the world are working feverishly toward better treatments for fibromyalgia, ones that target several symptoms at once with few side effects. As of right now, there are no medications specifically approved by the U.S. Food and Drug Administration to treat fibromyalgia. There is hope, however, that that will change in the next few years as researchers forge ahead with their experiments on treatments for fibromyalgia. Some of these are even entering the final stages of clinical trials as this book goes to press. In any case, it appears that someday soon, fibro sufferers will have more treatment options at their disposal.

Milnacipran

Milnacipran is the first in a new class of antidepressants known as norepinephrine serotonin reuptake inhibitors (NSRIs) and is currently used as an antidepressant by 3 million people around the world. These medications work by blocking the reuptake of both norepinephrine and serotonin, neurotransmitters involved in regulating mood and pain. It's believed that people with fibromyalgia do not have enough norepinephrine and serotonin, which results in depression and chronic pain.

Fact

On average, a new drug takes twelve years to go from preclinical testing to approval. The earliest phases begin with tests done on lab animals, then testing progresses through three phases of clinical trials before reaching the review process at the FDA. Even the review process takes about two and a half years.

In phase two clinical trials by the pharmaceutical company Cypress Bioscience, Inc., fibro patients who took milnacipran experienced significant improvements in their pain and fatigue symptoms. They also reported less depression. The study also found that most patients were able to take high dosages without problems. The most common side effect was nausea, but most problems were mild or moderate in intensity.

The drug is now in phase three of clinical trials, the last phase before FDA approval. Cypress Bioscience has made it the company's goal to be the first to market a product in the United States specifically for the treatment of fibromyalgia. The company hopes to submit a new drug application to the FDA by late 2006 at the earliest.

Pyridostigmine

People who have fibromyalgia generally have low levels of human growth hormone (HGH), the lack of which causes poor health. They tend to be overweight and have low energy, impaired thinking, and mild depression. They also have poor tolerance for cold temperatures and low blood volume. Many of these symptoms of low HGH overlap with those in fibromyalgia.

But treating people with HGH is unrealistic. Although HGH does produce a positive response in most patients, treatment takes at least six months for results and currently costs about $80,000 a year, which most insurance companies won't cover. That's why some researchers are considering the use of pyridostigmine, which can influence the production of HGH during exercise. Pyridostigmine (Mestinon) is currently used to treat myasthenia gravis, an autoimmune neuromuscular disease in which the patient's muscles become weakened.

Normal healthy people secrete growth hormone during sleep and after they exercise. But a study by Robert Bennett, MD, in 2002, found that people who had fibromyalgia did not produce as much human growth hormone in response to exercise. When the subjects were tested a month later and given pyridostigmine, HGH levels increased eightfold after exercise.

Pyridostigmine is believed to work by inhibiting somatostatin, a hormone that occurs in abundance in people with fibromyalgia and inhibits growth hormone. By giving the drug to people before exercise—and thus blocking somatostatin from inhibiting growth hormone—the subjects had more growth hormone following exercise. Growth hormone is needed to regenerate tissues and repair muscles after exercise, which would definitely benefit people with fibromyalgia.

To better understand the effects of pyridostigmine, researchers at the Oregon School of Nursing Research are examining the effects of pyridostigmine on women during exercise. The study will be done over a six-month period and will measure the impact of pyridostigmine on fibro pain.

Xyrem

Sodium oxybate (Xyrem) has had a checkered history, but it is emerging as a possible treatment for fibromyalgia. Xyrem is a central nervous system depressant and a form of gamma hydroxybutyrate (GHB), a naturally occurring metabolite. In the 1980s, GHB was popular among body builders, who used it to reduce fat and build muscle. It was also abused as a recreational drug and involved in several reported incidences of date rape. After several adverse events, including death, the FDA removed GHB from store shelves.

Subsequent research by a company called Orphan Medical soon discovered that Xyrem was effective in reducing cataplexy attacks in people with narcolepsy, a sleep disorder characterized by excessive daytime sleepiness. Cataplexy is a condition in which muscles become suddenly weak or paralyzed during intense emotional reactions, such as laughter, anger, or fear.

Other researchers soon learned that Xyrem could reduce the symptoms of fibromyalgia. In studies with fibromyalgia patients, Xyrem decreased the intrusion of alpha waves during sleep and increased REM sleep. In addition, Xyrem reduced pain and fatigue in the patients. Buoyed by these findings, Orphan did a follow-up trial, which was completed in 2005. Results were not available at the time of this publication.

Because of its history of abuse and adverse events, access to Xyrem is highly restricted. At this time, the drug is available only through the Xyrem Central Pharmacy, which is run by the makers of the drug, Orphan Medical. Xyrem is a federally controlled substance approved for medical use only.

High-Dose Mirapex

People who have Parkinson's disease are slowly losing a chemical in their brains called dopamine, which controls muscle function. As a result, patients typically suffer from tremors, or involuntary shaking of the limbs. In some cases, muscles become stiff and rigid, and movement becomes quite slow.

One of the drugs used to treat Parkinson's is pramipexole (Mirapex), a dopamine agonist that mimics the action of real dopamine. In addition, Mirapex is used in low doses to treat restless legs syndrome. Researchers recently learned that Mirapex may also help relieve symptoms of fibromyalgia.

A double-blind placebo-controlled study involved forty-nine patients with fibromyalgia. Those who were given pramipexole used a gradual escalating dose of Mirapex over a fourteen-week period.

The dosage started at 0.25 mg the first week and ended at 4.5 mg during the final three weeks. By the end of the study, most patients in the group who took Mirapex experienced improvements in pain, fatigue, and function. The drug caused few side effects, with the most common being nausea and weight loss. More research into Mirapex and fibromyalgia are expected.

Question

What is a double-blind placebo-controlled study?
This type of study is considered the gold standard of research, in which neither the researchers nor the subjects know who receives the treatment and who receives the placebo. The arrangement is designed to avoid bias in the research process.

Revolutionary Treatments

Because fibromyalgia is so complex, not everyone agrees on how to best treat it. Conventional doctors may treat it simply with antidepressants, muscle relaxants, and a careful balance of rest and exercise. But some doctors are taking bolder steps and attempting treatments that others might consider cutting edge.

One problem in treating fibromyalgia is that the disease is still not well understood. No one knows why the body becomes hypersensitive to pain or why it falls prey to fatigue. And it's still a mystery as to whether poor sleep is the cause or the result of fibromyalgia.

More and more, researchers are beginning to suspect that fibromyalgia is not the result of one problem but actually the consequence of several different dysfunctions in the body. In fact, it's even possible that FMS is more than one disease. So while one person may experience fibromyalgia as the result of a thyroid problem, another may develop it because of candida overgrowth. Different causes of fibromyalgia would certainly help explain the diversity of symptoms and why different patients respond to different treatments. These schools of thought have resulted in various modes of treatment. Some doctors may consider these treatments revolutionary. But others have incorporated them into their practice.

Adrenal Depletion

Many people who develop fibromyalgia are high-strung, Type-A personalities, who are driven, highly motivated workaholics vulnerable to stress. Having fibromyalgia only worsens their stress.

One theory of fibromyalgia—which applies especially to those who have fatigue as their primary symptom—is that it stems from adrenal depletion or exhaustion. Adrenal depletion occurs in people with overactive sympathetic nervous systems. The sympathetic nervous system is the part of the autonomic nervous system that responds to danger, stress, and excitement by increasing heartbeat and blood pressure. When it's overactive, the adrenal glands are taxed. As a result, these little thumb-sized glands—which are located on top of your kidneys—constantly churn out cortisol and adrenaline, the two stress hormones. In people who are overly stressed, do too much, or skip meals, blood sugar levels dip. The body releases cortisol, which then causes the liver to release glycogen (sugar or energy) stored in its reserves.

Eventually, if the stress persists, the prolonged demand for cortisol depletes the adrenal gland's ability to make it. If the adrenals can't make enough cortisol, your blood sugar will drop to the point where the backup system kicks in and your body starts to release adrenaline. As a result of this adrenal activity and low blood sugar, you may experience extreme fatigue, anxiety, and heart palpitations. You may be irritable and experience lightheadedness upon standing. You may also lose weight without even trying.

Diagnosing and Treating Adrenal Depletion

Most patients who have adrenal depletion tend to be thin and fatigued. But to figure out if you are suffering from adrenal depletion, your doctor may do a blood test to measure adrenal hormones.

Blood tests may also reveal abnormally high levels of potassium and low levels of sodium, which can result from adrenal depletion.

Treatment usually involves low doses of cortisol, in amounts below what the body normally produces. Most patients will respond well and feel less fatigued. Treatment may also require stress reduction strategies, eating more frequently, and eating more complex carbohydrates and salt, which can restore proper electrolyte balance. Some patients are also treated with licorice root extract or adrenal support supplements, such as vitamin C, the B vitamins, and certain amino acids.

Candida Hypersensitivity Syndrome

The natural world has more than 1,000 types of yeast. In the human body, yeast inhabits the skin, the digestive tract, and the vagina, where its numbers are kept in check by our immune system, healthy bacteria (called probiotics), and the intact membrane of the digestive tract. The predominant disease-causing kind of yeast that lives in humans is called candida albicans.

It is believed that in some people, candida albicans proliferates when our natural defenses break down. Sometimes, the extended use of antibiotics can spur the growth of candida. Eating a diet high in sugar also appears to contribute. The yeast grows out of control, seeps into the blood, and sets the immune system into action. When white blood cells and immunoglobulins attack the yeast in the gut, chemicals are released into the blood, causing a spate of health problems.

Symptoms of yeast overgrowth mimic those of fibromyalgia. In people who have fibromyalgia, yeast overgrowth may cause symptoms of hypothyroidism—even though traditional thyroid tests are normal. Chemicals released by the yeast get absorbed into the body and disrupt the normal function of thyroid hormone by inhibiting the alpha thyroid receptor, which is found in skin, muscles, bones, connective tissues, and certain parts of the brain.

Question

Why can't blood tests detect hypothyroidism caused by candida hypersensitivity?
There are different types of receptors for thyroid hormone. The receptor that determines the amount of hormone in the blood is not affected by yeast overgrowth, so blood tests appear normal. But the receptors in skin, muscles, bones, connective tissue, and certain parts of the brain are affected by excess candida. Since the toxins responsible haven't yet been identified, they can't be measured in the blood.

In healthy people, thyroid hormone works by stimulating the production of metabolic enzymes that produce energy and blocking excess production of substance P, which makes you sensitive to pain. But in people with fibromyalgia, whose alpha receptor has been inhibited, the levels of metabolic enzymes decrease, and levels of substance P increase. The result is the fatigue and pain associated with fibromyalgia. In addition, the yeast releases a substance called tartaric acid, which may inhibit metabolism of lactic acid, thereby aggravating fatigue.

The connection between yeast hypersensitivity and fibromyalgia is highly controversial. Not every physician believes it exists. But at Fibromyalgia Treatment Centers of America in Chicago, where Dr. Michael McNett treats fibro patients for candida, 70 percent of his patients test positive for candida hypersensitivity syndrome. When patients are treated for candida overgrowth, 75 percent of them experience at least a 25 percent improvement in their fibromyalgia symptoms. And in approximately an eighth of his patients, the symptoms of fibro disappear.

Diagnosing and Treating Candida Hypersensitivity

There are a number of tests available for candida hypersensitivity syndrome, but most are highly unreliable, including anticandida antibodies, stool candida counts, and skin tests for candida allergy. One test that does appear to be an accurate measure is a blood test for antibodies attached to a piece of the candida cell wall. You can also find a simple questionnaire at the Yeast Connection Web site (*www.yeastconnection.com*).

If you do have yeast overgrowth, your doctor will recommend a diet low in refined carbs. You may also be given antifungal medication, such as nystatin, and acidophilus, a probiotic commonly found in yogurt. Treatment usually lasts six months.

Peripheral Thyroid Resistance

It's a fact that many patients with fibromyalgia have symptoms similar to those who suffer from hypothyroidism. Yet thyroid tests on most people with FMS reveal that their thyroid levels are normal.

But some experts believe that the underlying cause of FMS is a problem called peripheral thyroid resistance. Studies by Dr. John Lowe have found that as many as 40 percent of all fibro patients have peripheral tissue resistance to thyroid hormone. To support the connection between thyroid resistance and fibromyalgia, they point to the many fibro patients who have been successfully treated with the same treatments used for hypothyroidism.

 Fact

One result of peripheral thyroid resistance is hypometabolism, in which your body's metabolism becomes abnormally slow. As a result, body temperature falls, and you may be prone to weight gain. Hypometabolism can also develop in people who have a sedentary lifestyle and in those with certain nutritional deficiencies.

In order to understand peripheral thyroid resistance, it helps to understand how a healthy thyroid works in conjunction with the pituitary gland. Every cell in our body depends on two thyroid hormones,

T3 and T4, for regulation of metabolism. When blood levels of T3 and T4 fall, the pituitary gland produces thyroid-stimulating hormone (TSH), which signals the thyroid to produce more T3 and T4. Once the blood levels of T3 and T4 increase, the pituitary decreases its TSH production.

In people who have peripheral thyroid resistance, cells lose the ability to recognize thyroid hormone and become resistant to normal thyroid hormones in the blood. The cause of this resistance remains a mystery. So even though the communication between the pituitary gland and the thyroid is normal, and the amount of thyroid hormone in the blood is perfectly normal, resistance to the hormones slows metabolism in the peripheral body tissues. The result can be fibromyalgia or other conditions that resemble hypothyroidism.

Diagnosing and Treating Peripheral Thyroid Resistance

It isn't easy to determine whether a patient has peripheral thyroid resistance, especially since blood tests will reveal that thyroid hormone and TSH levels are normal. Often, in fact, the only way to know for sure is to treat the patient with progressively larger doses of T3.

When patients are treated with high dosages of T3, the TSH levels drop precipitously. Many physicians may find these low levels alarming, but they are not typically harmful if the dosage is raised slowly and the patient is closely monitored. Treatment will then reveal whether a patient did indeed have peripheral thyroid resistance. Those who have it will notice a significant reduction in their symptoms. Those who do not, however, may develop a condition called thyrotoxicosis, or severe hyperthyroidism. Thyrotoxicosis can be dangerous, which is why any patient who undergoes this treatment must be closely monitored.

Chiari Malformation and Cervical Stenosis

Some experts wonder whether malformations of the brain might be the cause behind the symptoms of fibromyalgia. Scientists are particularly intrigued by Chiari malformation and cervical stenosis. In people with Chiari malformation, the cerebellum protrudes through the bottom of the skull into the spinal canal, compressing the spinal cord and causing poor circulation of cerebrospinal fluid between the spinal cord and the brain. Cervical stenosis occurs when the spinal canal is too narrow for the spinal cord and presses on it. Symptoms of Chiari malformation and cervical stenosis, which may resemble those of fibromyalgia, include pain, fatigue, headaches, dizziness, and difficulties with cognitive function. Like fibromyalgia, Chiari often is not evident until a head or neck injury is sustained.

In recent years, many patients diagnosed with fibromyalgia have found relief from their symptoms after surgeries to correct Chiari malformation or cervical stenosis. The surgery has also relieved dizziness, pain, headaches, poor sleep, and numbness. In addition, it has alleviated irritable bowel syndrome, memory or cognitive problems, vision difficulties, weakness, and fatigue.

Although surgeons have been correcting Chiari malformations and cervical stenosis for many decades, the connection between these conditions and fibromyalgia is relatively new and fairly controversial. Some members of the medical community now recommend MRIs and neurological tests for people diagnosed with fibromyalgia. But critics say the surgery provides false hope to fibro sufferers desperate for relief.

Whether fibromyalgia is always—or ever—the result of Chiari malformation or cervical stenosis is uncertain. It's also unclear whether surgery can always benefit people with fibromyalgia. But based on the success of many patients, the link between fibromyalgia and Chiari malformation and cervical stenosis certainly warrants more research and consideration.

Diagnosing and Treating Chiari Malformation

To determine whether you have Chiari malformation or cervical stenosis, you will need an MRI of your brain, the base of your skull, and the spinal cord. Your doctor may recommend an MRI if you have overactive reflexes of the arms and a general lack of coordination.

If a deformity or malformation is detected, your doctor may recommend surgery. However, not every patient requires surgery to treat these deformities. Some people may achieve relief by wearing a neck brace. Others may benefit from short-term steroid treatment. Postural training can also help reduce the pain.

Guaifenesin

Most people know guaifenesin as the main ingredient in the cough syrup Robitussin, where it is used to loosen mucus. For years, Dr. R. Paul St. Armand has recommended guaifenesin as a treatment for fibromyalgia. The drug is believed to work by promoting the excretion of phosphate through the urine and ridding body tissue of harmful phosphate deposits.

But the treatment has been fraught with controversy. The only valid study ever done, which was conducted by Robert Bennett, found no difference between women with fibromyalgia who took guaifenesin and those who took a placebo. The study also found no evidence that guaifenesin promotes the excretion of uric acid and no indication that phosphate excretion helps relieve fibromyalgia. Still, a significant number of fibro patients have had success using guaifenesin, which is why the subject deserves more research and study. The key may be to first identify patients who excrete low amounts of phosphate in their urine and to then treat them with guaifenesin.

Subclinical Infections

Days before you develop the first signs of a cold, you feel fine. You're energetic, busy, and appear perfectly well. You don't feel bad until the cold actually strikes. In reality, however, the infection was lingering in your body for some time before any symptoms first appeared. That's a subclinical infection.

It's possible that people who have fibromyalgia are living with a subclinical infection, or even several at a time. The infection could be lurking in body tissue and cells and wreaking havoc with the body's immune system.

Infections have already been found to play a role in illnesses such as HIV-AIDS and some autoimmune diseases. Researchers have found evidence of many types of infection in the blood of people with fibromyalgia, among them mycoplasma, Chlamydia, Lyme, and HHV-6. These findings suggest that these microorganisms may play a role in causing the symptoms of CFIDs and fibro.

Although these agents may not be the sole cause of fibromyalgia, their presence certainly warrants more research and attention. Treating these infections could in some cases reduce or even eliminate the symptoms.

The Importance of Retrograde Research

Why does one fibromyalgia patient recover while another suffers endlessly for years and years? What kind of treatments does a successful patient use? Why does one treatment work for one patient and not for another? Such baffling questions could be answered if more retrograde research was done.

Retrograde research would involve bringing together hundreds, perhaps thousands of patients who have stopped having symptoms of fibromyalgia. Researchers would then gather information and details about the remedies they used to get better. To pinpoint the beneficial treatments, patients would have to eliminate different therapies and see which ones brought back the symptoms of fibromyalgia. The research would then help scientists identify the different subtypes of fibromyalgia and the common mechanism that produces symptoms. It would also help determine specific treatments that work on different symptoms.

Toward a Better Understanding

Pain. Fatigue. Sleep problems. What is the connection between this triad of symptoms? Does the pain cause the fatigue? Or does fatigue cause pain? Is poor sleep a symptom of fibromyalgia? Or a result of it? Or, more likely, is there some common underlying mechanism that gives rise to all three? Answers to these questions could help provide a better understanding of fibromyalgia.

Clearly, a lot of research has been done on the pain of fibromyalgia. But people who develop fibromyalgia don't just develop pain.

Most also develop fatigue and sleep disorders, as well as Raynaud's phenomenon, irritable bowel and/or bladder, tremors, tingling/numbness, and difficulty with thinking and memory. Whatever is causing their pain must also be related to these other conditions.

Fact

A study funded by the National Institute of Arthritis and Musculoskeletal and Skin Diseases has found that fibromyalgia seems to have more of a genetic connection than rheumatoid arthritis (RA). As compared to RA, family members of people with fibro were more likely to also have fibro. The research raises the prospect of a genetic link in fibromyalgia.

As researchers look deeper into the mechanisms that affect all three primary symptoms, they will be pinpointing the factors at the root of fibro. Hopefully, that will guide them toward medications that will someday cure the illness, not just cover up symptoms.

Should You Assist in Research?

Before a treatment receives approval from the U.S. Food and Drug Administration, it requires several research studies to prove that the treatment is safe and effective. That's where clinical trials come in.

Clinical trials, also called clinical studies, are carefully conducted research studies performed using human volunteers in order to answer specific questions about a treatment or therapy. The treatment might be a new vaccine, drug, medical device, or procedure. The trials are done after research in laboratories shows promising results in animals.

The goal of these trials is to find out how the new therapy or procedure will work in people and to determine its risks and its effectiveness. Clinical trials also look at methods that prevent, diagnose, and screen disease. They may also uncover ways to improve quality of life for patients.

Several different kinds of organizations are involved in doing clinical trials, including doctors, medical institutions, pharmaceutical companies, foundations, government agencies, and others. The trials are done in various settings, ranging from a small doctor's office to a large university setting or hospital. All research is overseen by an institutional review board made up of an independent committee of physicians, community advocates, and others who oversee the ethics of the research. The board also ensures that the rights of the participants are protected and reviews the research on a periodic basis.

As a person with fibromyalgia, you might consider participating in a clinical trial of a treatment or procedure for fibromyalgia. Perhaps you've exhausted your options and want to try something different. Or maybe you have the altruistic desire to contribute to science. In any case, a clinical trial may be something to consider. At press time, there were twenty-four trials recruiting patients who have fibromyalgia or related symptoms.

By participating in a research study, you might gain access to a medication that is not widely available. You may also enjoy medical care at leading health-care facilities. Before you can participate, however, you have to make sure you qualify for the trial. Some people may be excluded because of age, gender, stage of disease, and other medical conditions. Some trials want candidates who have a certain condition. Others might require that you stop all your other medications, something your condition may not allow you to do.

 Alert

Some health-care professionals receive compensation for referring or enrolling patients in clinical trials. The U.S. Food and Drug Administration considers this a potential conflict of interest. While your health-care provider may not necessarily share this information with you, you may want to ask whether she—or any of the investigators on the trial—has a vested interest in the trial.

After meeting with the doctors and nurses involved in the trial, you will need to sign an informed consent document that says you understand the risks and benefits of participating. Being part of a clinical trial does involve risks. Some participants might be given a placebo, or inactive treatment. Those who are treated may experience unpleasant, even life-threatening side effects. You may also have to endure frequent visits to the testing site and hospital stays. And for all the time and energy you invest, you may also find that the treatment has no beneficial effect on your health.

Before deciding, check out the Web site *www.clinicaltrials.gov*, where you will find a list of trials and questions to consider. Discuss the process with your physician, family members, and friends. Balance the positives with the negatives and gather information about specific trials. You might also contact doctors, hospitals, or health-care organizations for information.

A Final Note

Research into fibromyalgia is ongoing and offers hope for a better understanding of the condition, more treatments, and perhaps someday a cure. Although the condition has been around for ages, our understanding of it is only now beginning to take off. For now, focus on your day-to-day challenges, and put forth your best effort in taking care of yourself. No matter what science turns up, you are your own best ally in caring for your health.

Organizations and Support Groups

Advocates for Fibromyalgia Funding, Treatment, Education and Research
P.O. Box 768
Libertyville, IL 60048-0768
Phone: 1-847-362-7807
Fax: 1-847-680-3922
www.affter.org

Fibromyalgia Network
P.O. Box 31750
Tucson, AZ 85751
Phone: 1-800-853-2929
www.fmnetnews.com

Fibromyalgia Support Network
c/o Global Healing Center
2040 North Loop West, Ste. 108
Houston, TX 77018
www.fibromyalgia-support.org

National Fibromyalgia Association
2200 N. Glassell St., Suite A
Orange, CA 92865
Phone: 1-714-921-0150
www.fmaware.org

National Fibromyalgia Partnership, Inc.
P.O. Box 160
Linden, VA 22642-0160
Phone: 1-866-725-4404
www.fmpartnership.org

National Fibromyalgia Research Association
P.O. Box 500
Salem, OR 97308
www.nfra.net

Oregon Fibromyalgia Foundation
120 NW 9th Avenue, Suite 216
Portland, OR 97209
www.myalgia.com

Other Organizations of Interest

American College of Rheumatology
1800 Century Place, Suite 250
Atlanta, GA 30345-4300
Phone: 1-404-633-3777
Fax: 1-404-633-1870
✑*www.rheumatology.org*

Arthritis Foundation
P.O. Box 7669
Atlanta, GA 30357-0669
1-800-283-7800
✑*www.arthritis.org*

The CFIDS Association of America
P.O. Box 220398
Charlotte, NC 28222-0398
Phone: 1-704-365-2343
✑*www.cfids.org*

National Center for Complementary and Alternative Medicine
National Institutes of Health
P.O. Box 7923
Gaithersburg, MD 20898-7923
Phone: 1-888-644-6226
Fax: 1-866-464-3616
✑*www.nccam.nih.gov*

National Institute of Arthritis and Musculoskeletal and Skin Diseases
1 AMS Circle
Bethesda, MD 20892-3675
Phone: 1-877-226-4267
Fax: 301-718-6366
✑*www.niams.nih.gov*

Social Security Administration
Office of Public Inquiries
Windsor Park Building
6401 Security Blvd.
Baltimore, MD 21325
Phone: 1-800-772-1213
✑*www.ssa.gov/disability*

Glossary

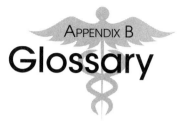

Acupuncture

A traditional Chinese medicine that involves the use of needles to restore the flow of energy in the body to promote health.

Adenosine triphosphate (ATP)

The body's primary source of fuel, produced in the mitochondria of body cells.

Adrenal depletion

A condition in which the adrenal glands fail to produce enough stress hormones, causing extreme exhaustion.

Adrenaline

A stress hormone that occurs in higher-than-normal levels in people with fibromyalgia.

Allodynia

A condition in which normally bearable sensations become painful.

Alpha-EEG anomaly

A sleep disorder characterized by the intrusion of alpha waves during stages of deep sleep. Alpha waves are associated with a state of being awake but relaxed.

Americans with Disabilities Act (ADA)

A law that prohibits employers with fifteen or more employees from discriminating against people with disabilities in decisions about hiring and employment.

Analgesics

Drugs that relieve pain. They may be narcotic or non-narcotic.

Anticonvulsants

Medications used to treat neuropathic pain that can sometimes treat fibromyalgia pain.

Autonomic nervous system

The part of the nervous system that regulates involuntary bodily functions and processes.

Benzodiazepines

A class of drugs that work as both antianxiety and antidepressant medications.

Biofeedback

A form of alternative therapy that trains the mind to control physical responses as measured on special instruments.

Botulinum A (Botox)

A drug that can be injected to paralyze the muscles that cause painful spasms in fibromyalgia.

Bruxism

Grinding and clenching of the teeth at night, often caused by stress, that may lead to TMJ.

Candida hypersensitivity syndrome

A condition caused by the overgrowth of candida albicans, a yeast.

Capsaicin

A substance in hot chili peppers that is used in topical creams.

Central nervous system

The part of the nervous system that includes the brain and spine.

Central sensitization

A condition resulting from stimulation of the pain fibers that is overly intense or goes on for too long.

Cervical stenosis

A condition that occurs when the spinal canal is too narrow for the spinal cord.

C-fiber

Slow-moving nerve fibers that are highly sensitive to chemical, mechanical, or thermal energy.

Chiari malformation

A condition in which the cerebellum protrudes through the bottom of the skull into the spinal canal, causing poor circulation of cerebrospinal fluid from the brain to the spinal cord.

Chiropractics

A medical treatment that involves realigning the spine to bring about healing.

Chronic fatigue immune deficiency syndrome (CFIDS)

A condition characterized by severe fatigue that has lasted six months or more.

Chronic myofascial pain

Persistent muscle pain associated with small spastic knots in the muscles.

Clinical trials

Research done in human volunteers to determine the efficacy of medications, surgeries, devices, or procedures.

Complementary and alternative medicine (CAM)

Therapies that are not considered mainstream in Western medicine and that are used alongside conventional therapies.

Cortisol

A stress hormone that occurs in higher than normal levels in people with fibromyalgia.

Cytokines

Proteins produced by white blood cells that help regulate immune function and which are elevated in people with CFIDs.

Deep tissue massage

A vigorous form of massage designed to loosen inflexible muscles.

Depression

A mood disorder characterized by extreme sadness that is common in fibromyalgia.

Endocrinologists

Medical doctors who specialize in treating the body's endocrine system, which regulates hormones.

Endorphins

Substances produced by the body that can help relieve pain and promote a feel-good response.

Fibro fog

A term that refers to the cognitive dysfunctions caused by fibromyalgia, including problems with memory and concentration.

Fibromyalgia

A medical syndrome characterized by widespread pain, sleep disturbance, and tender points around the body.

Guaifenesin

A cough-syrup ingredient that is sometimes used to treat fibromyalgia.

Guided imagery

The use of positive images to promote good health.

HPA axis

The hypothalamic-pituitary-adrenal axis, which is involved in releasing hormones that aid in the process of coping with stress.

Growth hormone

A hormone responsible for repairing muscles that is reduced in people with fibromyalgia.

Hyperalgesia

A condition in which mildly painful events become very painful.

Hypothyroidism

A condition in which the thyroid gland fails to produce enough thyroid hormone, causing fatigue. The condition resembles fibromyalgia and may also coexist with it.

Interstitial cystitis

Chronic hyperactivity of the bladder that can cause discomfort and pain in the bladder and surrounding pelvic region.

Irritable bowel syndrome

A chronic gastrointestinal condition characterized by cramps, abdominal pain, bloating, constipation, and diarrhea, common in fibromyalgia sufferers.

Lidocaine

A local anesthesia used in injections for fibro pain relief.

Lupus

An autoimmune disorder characterized by fatigue, painful joints,
rash, and fever that may resemble
or coexist with fibromyalgia.

Lyme disease

A bacterial disease transmitted
by ticks that can cause symptoms
that resemble fibromyalgia or may
trigger FMS.

Massage

The manual manipulation of soft
body tissues to promote relaxation, increase blood flow, and
reduce muscle tension.

Milnacipran

The first in a new class of antidepressants, known as norepinephrine serotonin reuptake inhibitors
(NSRIs), being researched as a
new drug for treatment of fibromyalgia.

Mixed reuptake inhibitor

Antidepressants that work by
balancing the amounts of the
neurotransmitters   serotonin,
dopamine, and norepinephrine.

Monoamine oxidase inhibitors

An older class of antidepressants,
used less often these days due to
side effects.

Multiple chemical sensitivities

Hypersensitivity to smells, noises,
and chemicals in the surrounding environment. Also called

idiopathic environmental intolerances.

Multiple sclerosis

An autoimmune disorder in which
the body attacks the nervous system, causing varying neurological
problems.

Myofascial release

A form of massage designed to
relieve tightness and restricted
movement in the fibrous or connective tissue.

Narcotics

Painkilling drugs derived from the
poppy plant that interfere with the
receptors in the body that transmit pain.

Neurologist

A medical doctor who specializes
in diagnosing, treating, and managing disorders of the brain and
nervous system.

Nociceptors

Receptors at the end of nerve
fibers that detect actual or potential tissue damage.

**Nonsteroidal anti-inflammatory drugs
(NSAIDs)**

A category of analgesics that alleviate pain by reducing inflammation.

Occupational therapist

A health-care professional who
helps patients learn new ways

of movement that minimize pain and strain.

Osteoarthritis

A degenerative condition in which the cartilage cushioning bones is eroded.

Osteopathic physicians

A health-care practitioner trained in osteopathy, a health science that places greater emphasis on treating the whole body and that stresses prevention and health maintenance.

Peripheral thyroid resistance

A condition in which body tissue becomes resistant to thyroid hormones.

Periodic limb movements during sleep

A condition characterized by purposeless maneuvers of the legs and feet during sleep.

Peripheral nervous system

An elaborate network of nerve fibers that receives information from inside and outside the body and then relays it to the brain.

Pharmacologist

Pharmacy-trained professionals who specialize in helping patients who take numerous or unusual medications.

Physiatrist

A doctor who specializes in physical medicine and works to restore function in injured muscles and joints.

Physical therapist

A health-care professional who helps patients cope with pain or recover from illness or surgery.

Placebo effect

A phenomenon in which healing is brought about simply by the patient's belief that a treatment will work.

Polymyalgia rheumatica

An arthritic condition caused by inflammation triggered by the immune system.

Pramipexole (Mirapex)

A drug used to treat Parkinson's and restless legs syndrome that is being studied as a treatment for fibromyalgia.

Pyridostigmine (Mestinon)

A treatment for myasthenia gravis that is being studied as a drug for treatment of fibromyalgia.

Raynaud's phenomenon

Vasospasms of the blood vessels in the extremities that causes coldness in the fingers, toes, and tips of the ears or nose.

Reiki

A Japanese treatment that uses the channeling of energy to promote healing.

Restless legs syndrome

A condition that typically occurs at night and makes the legs feel twitchy, uneasy, and tingly. It is common in fibro patients.

Retrograde research

The study of patients who have recovered from an illness to determine what helped in their recovery.

Rheumatic disease

Conditions characterized by inflammation in muscles, joints, and fibrous tissue. People with rheumatic illnesses are at greater risk for fibromyalgia.

Rheumatoid arthritis

An autoimmune disease characterized by inflammation of the joints that may resemble or coexist with fibromyalgia.

Rheumatologist

A doctor who specializes in the diagnosis, treatment, and care of autoimmune disorders.

Selective serotonin reuptake inhibitors (SSRIs)

A newer category of antidepressants that work by blocking the removal of serotonin.

Sensory somatic nervous system

The part of the nervous system responsible for voluntary and involuntary movement in response to external stimuli.

Serotonin

A neurotransmitter involved in regulating pain and mood that is deficient in fibromyalgia patients.

Sleep apnea

A condition in which breathing is temporarily obstructed during sleep, causing poor sleep quality.

Social Security Disability Insurance (SSDI)

A type of financial assistance provided by the Social Security Administration for workers under the age of sixty-five who can no longer work or who have lost income due to disability.

Sodium oxybate (Xyrem)

A drug used to treat a form of narcolepsy that is being studied as a treatment for fibromyalgia.

Somatostatin

A hormone that occurs in abundance in people with fibromyalgia and that inhibits growth hormone.

Substance P

A chemical that increases your nerves' sensitivity to pain and that is found in higher levels in the spinal fluid of people with FMS.

Supplemental Security Income (SSI)

A form of financial assistance from the Social Security Administration for disabled people who have limited income and who may not have worked in the past.

Swedish massage

A gentle form of massage that does not use much pressure on body tissues.

Temporomandibular joint disorder (TMJ)

A condition affecting the joint connecting the lower and upper jaws that can cause stiffness, headaches, and clicking noises. It is common in people with fibromyalgia.

Tender points

Places located around the body that are used to monitor pain sensitivity and to help diagnose fibromyalgia.

Tricyclic antidepressants

Medications for depression that have been used to treat fibromyalgia by restoring chemical imbalances and inducing sleep.

Trigger point

A small spastic knot that causes local pain but can also send or refer pain to other parts of the body.

Trigger-point therapy

A treatment that involves stretching and deep manual pressure to relax knotted muscles and relieve pain.

Vulvodynia

Chronic pain or discomfort of the vulva, or external female genitalia.

Wind-up phenomenon

A significant increase in your response to pain caused by central sensitization.

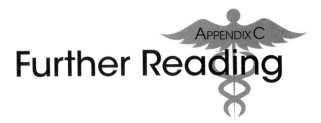

Further Reading

Books

Adamson, Eve. *The Everything Stress Management Book* (Avon, MA: Adams Media, 2002).

The Arthritis Foundation's Guide to Good Living with Fibromyalgia (Atlanta, GA: Arthritis Foundation, 2001).

Balch, James F., and Stengler, Mark. *Prescription for Natural Cures* (Hoboken, NJ: John Wiley & Sons, Inc., 2004).

Burton, Gail. *Candida, The Silent Epidemic* (Fairfield, CT: Asian Publishing, 2003).

Crook, William. *The Yeast Connection Handbook* (New York: Random House, 1986).

Davies, Clair. *The Trigger Point Therapy Workbook* (Oakland, CA: New Harbinger Publications, 2004).

Davis, Laura. *Allies in Healing* (New York, NY: Harper Collins, 1991).

Duyff, Roberta Larson. *American Dietetic Association Complete Food and Nutrition Guide* (Hoboken, NJ: John Wiley & Sons, 2002).

Fischer, Harry D., and Yu, Winnie. *What to Do When the Doctor Says It's Rheumatoid Arthritis* (Gloucester, MA: Fair Winds Press, 2005).

Good Living with Fibromyalgia Workbook: Activities for a Better Life (Atlanta, GA: Arthritis Foundation, 2002).

Hammerly, Milton. Fibromyalgia: The New Integrative Approach (Avon, MA: Adams Media, 2000).

Kelly, Julie, and Devonshire, Rosalie. *Taking Charge of Fibromyalgia* (Wayzata, MN: Fibromyalgia Educational Systems, 2001).

Marek, Claudia Craig. *The First Year Fibromyalgia: An Essential Guide for the Newly Diagnosed* (New York: Marlowe & Co., 2003).

Matallana, Lynne. *The Complete Idiot's Guide to Fibromyalgia* (New York, NY: Alpha Books, 2005).

Pellegrino, Mark. *Fibromyalgia Up Close and Personal* (Columbus, OH: Anadem Publishing, 2005).

Salt, William, and Season, Edwin. *Fibromyalgia and the Mind Body Spirit Connection* (Columbus, OH: Parkview Publishing, 2000).

Shomon, Mary. *Living Well with Chronic Fatigue Syndrome and Fibromyalgia* (New York, NY: HarperCollins Publishers, 2004).

Siebert, Al. *The Resiliency Advantage* (San Francisco, CA: Berrett-Koehler Publishers, Inc., 2005).

Smolin, Lori A., and Grosvenor, Mary B. *Nutrition Science and Applications* (Orlando, FL: Saunders College Publishing, 1994).

Starlanyl, Devin, and Copeland, Mary Ellen. *Fibromyalgia and Chronic Myofascial Pain: A Survival Manual* (Oakland, CA: New Harbinger Publications, 2001).

Teitelbaum, Jacob. *From Fatigued to Fantastic* (New York, NY: Avery Books, 2001).

Wallace, Daniel J., and Wallace, Janice Brock. *Making Sense of Fibromyalgia* (New York: Oxford University Press, 1999).

Web Sites

American College of Sports Medicine
www.acsm.org
Articles and information on health, fitness, and exercise.

American Council on Exercise
www.acefitnes.org
Good site for information about health, fitness, and exercise.

American Council on Headache Education
www.achenet.org
An excellent source for information about treating and managing headaches.

ImmuneSupport.com
www.immunesupport.com
Articles and information for people with fibromyalgia and chronic fatigue syndrome.

Interstitial Cystitis Association
www.ic-help.org
Information about treatment and management of interstitial cystitis.

Irritable Bowel Self-Help Group
www.ibsgroup.org
On-line community for IBS sufferers, with articles on IBS.

The Lupus Foundation
✍*www.lupus.org*
An excellent source of
information about the
diagnosis, treatment, and
management of lupus.

National Sleep Foundation
✍*www.nof.org*
Articles and information about
sleep and sleep problems.

TMJ Association
✍*www.tmj.org*
An excellent source of
information about
temporomandibular joint
disorder.

Additional Helpful Web Sites

*American Academy of Family
Physicians*
✍*www.aafp.org*

American Academy of Osteopathy
✍*www.academyofosteopathy
.org*

*American Academy of Physical
Medicine and Rehabilitation*
✍*www.aapmr.org*

American College of Rheumatology
✍*www.rheumatology.org*

American Pain Foundation
✍*www.painfoundation.org*

American Psychiatric Association
✍*www.psych.org*

American Psychological Association
✍*www.apa.org*

CFIDS Association of America
✍*www.cfids.org*

ClinicalTrials.gov
✍*www.clinicaltrials.gov*

Cypress Bioscience Inc.
✍*www.cypressbio.com*

Dr.Lowe.com
✍*www.drlowe.com*

Fibromyalgia Network
✍*www.fmnetnews.com*

Fibromyalgia Support Network
✍*www.fibromyalgia-support
.org*

Fibromyalgia Syndrome Resource
✍*www.fibromyalgia-
symptoms.org*

MayoClinic.com
✍*www.mayoclinic.com*

Medicinenet.com
✍*www.medicinenet.com*

*National Center for Complementary
and Alternative Medicine*
✍*www.nccam.nih.gov*

National Fibromyalgia Association
✍*www.fmaware.org*

National Headache Foundation
✍*www.headaches.org*

*National Institute of Arthritis and
Musculoskeletal and Skin Diseases*
✍*www.niams.nih.gov*

National Institutes of Health
✍*www.nih.gov*

National Library of Medicine
✍*www.nlm.nih.gov*

National Safety Council
✍*www.nsc.org*

Nothing But Yoga
✍*www.nothingbutyoga.com*

Oregon Fibromyalgia Foundation
✍*www.myalgia.com*

Oregon Hypnotherapy Association
✍*www.hypnosis-oregon.com*

Social Security Administration
✍*www.ssa.gov*

Spine-Health.com
✍*www.spine-health.com*

*Tennessee Occupational Therapy
Association*
✍*www.tnota.org/focus_fibro.
html*

The Hormone Foundation
✍*www.hormone.org*

U.S. Food and Drug Administration
✍*www.fda.gov*

WebMD.com
✍*www.webmd.com*

Xyrem
✍*www.xyrem.com*

Electronic Articles

"A Perfect Posture Guide," article from First Choice Chiropractic, Ann Arbor, Michigan (*www.firstchoicechiropractic.com/PostureGuide.htm*).

"Annual survey shows Americans are working from many different locations outside their employer's office," press release from ITAC, the Telework Advisory Group for Worldatwork, Oct. 4, 2005 (*www.workingfromanywhere .org/news/pr100405.htm*).

"Position Statement on IEI," American Academy of Allergies, Asthma & Immunology (*www.aaaai.org/media/resources/academy_statements/ position_statements/ps35. asp*).

Dean, Carolyn. "Fibromyalgia, Chronic Fatigue and the Yeast Connection: Is Yeast the Missing Link?" (*www.mercola.com/2004/jul/31/fibromyalgia_yeast .htm*).

Environmental Protection Agency: Indoor Air Facts No. 4 (revised): Sick Building Syndrome (SBS) (*www.epa.gov/iaq/pubs/sbs.html*).

"Chronic Pain," Medicinenet.com (*www.medicinenet.com/chronic_pain/ article.htm*).

"Fibromyalgia, Chronic Fatigue Syndrome and Migraines," Michigan Head-Pain and Neurological Institute (*www.mhni.com/faqs_other_disorders .html#is*).

"Fibromyalgia: How is it treated?" Express Scripts' Drug Digest (*www. drugdigest.org*).

"Genital pain linked to increased pain sensitivity," University of Michigan Health Systems press release, August 2004 (*www.med.umich.edu/opm/ newspage/2004/vpain.htm*).

Graham, Rhonda. "The Purpose of Pain Scales," Aetna Intelihealth (*www .intelihealth.com/IH/ihtIH/WSIHW000/29721/32087.html#wong*).

"Fibromyalgia and Adrenal Hormones," Great Smokies Diagnostic Labs (*www.gsdl.com/home/assessments/finddisease/fibromyalgia/adrenal_ hormones.html*).

"Multiple Chemical Sensitivities," Ohio State University Extension Fact Sheet (*www.ohioline.osu.edu/cd-fact/0192.html*).

"Pain and the brain: Sex, hormones & genetics affect brain's pain control system, shaping a person's pain perception, U-M research finds," University of Michigan Health Systems, Feb. 18, 2003 (*www.med.umich.edu/opm/ newspage/2003/painbrain.htm*).

"Perfectionism Bad for Your Health," Medical Study News, June 2, 2004 (*www.news-medical.net*).

"Research-related tips to reduce exercise program dropout rate," American College of Sports Medicine press release, March 8, 2002 (*www.acsm.org/ publications/newsreleases2002/dropoutrate030702.htm*).

Preidt, Robert. "For many, work is a real pain," MedicineNet.com, July 13, 2005 (*www.medicinenet.com/script/main/art.asp?articlekey=52530*).

Schorr, Melissa. "Is it all in my head?" Psychology Today (May/June 2005): 70–78 (*http://cms.psychologytoday.com/articles/pto-20050503-000002.html*).

Shomon, Mary. "Candida and Yeast and the Connection to Thyroid Disease and Fibromyalgia: An Interview with Dr. Michael McNett" (*www.thyroid-info .com*).

"Stress at Work," National Institute of Occupational Safety and Health (*www .cdc.gov/niosh/stresswk.html*).

Wierenga, Dale E., and Eaton, C. Robert. "Phases of Product Development," Alliance Pharmaceutical Corp. (*www.allp.com/drug_dev.htm*).

Print Articles

Alvarez, David J., and Rockwell, Pamela G. "Trigger Points: Diagnosis and Management," *American Family Physician*, vol. 65 (Feb. 15, 2002): 653–60.

Bigatti, S. M., et al. "An examination of the physical health, health care use, and psychological well-being of spouses of people with fibromyalgia syndrome," *Health Psychology*, vol. 21 (March 2002): 157–66.

Bou-Holaigah, I., et al. "Provocation of hypotension and pain during upright tilt table testing in adults with fibromyalgia," *Clinical & Experimental Rheumatology*, vol. 15 (May–June 1997): 239–46.

Castro, I. "Prevalence of abuse in fibromyalgia and other rheumatic disorders at a specialized clinic in rheumatic diseases in Guatemala City," *Journal of Clinical Rheumatology*, vol. 11 (June 2005): 140–5.

Diatchenko, L., et al. "Genetic basis for individual variations in pain perception and the development of a chronic pain condition,"

Human Molecular Genetics, vol. 14 (Jan. 1, 2005): 135–43.

Dinerman, H., and Steere, A. C. "Lyme disease associated with fibromyalgia," *Annals of Internal Medicine,* vol. 117 (Aug. 15, 1992): 281–5.

Eisen, S. A., et al. "Gulf War veterans' health: medical evaluation of a U.S. cohort," *Annals of Internal Medicine,* vol. 142 (June 7, 2005): 881–90.

Finestone, H. M., et al. "Chronic pain and health care utilization in women with a history of childhood sexual abuse," *Child Abuse & Neglect,* vol. 24 (April 2000): 547–56.

Giesecke, J., et al. "Quantitative sensory testing in vulvodynia patients and increased peripheral pressure pain sensitivity," *Obstetrics and Gynecology,* vol. 104 (July 2004): 126–33.

Glass, J. M., et al. "Memory beliefs and function in fibromyalgia patients," *Journal of Psychosomatic Research,* vol. 58 (March 2005): 263–9.

Goldenberg, D., et al. "A randomized, double-blind crossover trial of fluoxetine and amitriptyline in the treatment of fibromyalgia," *Arthritis and Rheumatism,* vol. 39 (Nov. 1996): 1852–9.

Heffez, Daniel S., et al. "Clinical evidence for cervical myelopathy due to Chiari malformation and spinal stenosis in a non-randomized group of patients with the diagnosis of fibromyalgia," *European Spine Journal,* vol. 13 (Oct. 2004): 516–23.

Holman, Andrew, et al. "A randomized, double-blind, placebo-controlled trial of pramipexole, a dopamine agonist, in patients with fibromyalgia receiving concomitant medications," *Arthritis and Rheumatism,* vol. 52 (Aug. 2005): 2495–505.

"Hormones may place women at greater risk for facial pain," University of Washington, Seattle, press release, Jan. 29, 1997.

Kelly, Janis. "The significance of gender." *Fibromyalgia Aware,* vol. 4 (June–Sept. 2003): 25.

Merchant, R. E., et al. "A review of recent clinical trials of the nutritional supplement Chlorella pyrenoidosa in the treatment of fibromyalgia, hypertension, and ulcerative colitis," *Alternative Therapies in Health and Medicine,* vol. 7 (May–June, 2001): 79–91.

Molnar, Amy. "Drug used to treat Parkinson's Disease may be beneficial in treating fibromyalgia," American College of Rheumatology press release, Aug. 2005.

Muller, B., et al. "Impaired Action of Thyroid Hormone Associated with Smoking in Women with Hypothyroidism," *New England Journal of Medicine*, vol. 333 (Oct. 12, 1995): 964–969.

Niaura, R., et al. "Hostility, the metabolic syndrome, and incident coronary heart disease," *Health Psychology*, vol. 21 (Nov. 2002): 588–593.

Rubinstein, Joshua, et al. "Executive control of cognitive processes in task switching," Journal of Experimental Psychology: *Human Perception and Performance*, vol. 27 (August 2001): 763–797.

Scharf, M. B., et al. "The effects of sodium oxybate on clinical symptoms and sleep patterns in patients with fibromyalgia," *The Journal of Rheumatology*, vol. 20 (May 2003): 1070–4.

Siddiqui, I. A., et al. "Antioxidants of the Beverage Tea in Promotion of Human Health," *Antioxidants & Redox Signaling*, vol. 6 (June 2004): 571–582.

Smith, W. S., et al. "Spinal manipulative therapy is an independent risk factor for vertebral artery dissection," *Neurology*, vol. 60 (May 13, 2003): 1424–8.

Straub, T. A. "Endoscopic carpal tunnel release: A prospective analysis of factors associated with unsatisfactory results," *Arthroscopy*, vol. 15 (April 1999): 269–74.

Suarez, E. C. "C-reactive protein is associated with psychological risk factors of cardiovascular disease in apparently healthy adults," *Psychosomatic Medicine*, vol. 66 (Sept. 2004): 684–91.

Sverdup, B. "Use Less Cosmetics, Suffer Less from Fibromyalgia?" *Journal of Women's Health*, vol. 13 (March 2004): 187–194.

Tindle, H. A., et al. "Factors associated with the use of mind body therapies among United States adults with musculoskeletal pain," *Complementary Therapies in Medicine*, vol. 13 (Sept. 2005): 155–164.

Viner, R., and Hotopf, M. "Childhood predictors of self reported chronic fatigue syndrome/myalgic encephalomyelitis in adults: National birth cohort study," *British Medical Journal*, vol. 329 (Oct. 23, 2004): 329–941.

Wallace, Daniel. "The Nobel Prize: A Lifetime of Fibromyalgia," *Fibromyalgia Aware*, vol. 4 (June–Sept. 2003): 24.

Waylonis, G. W., et al. "A profile of fibromyalgia in occupational environments," *American Journal of Physical Medicine & Rehabilitation*, vol. 73 (April 1994): 112–5.

Index

A

acupuncture, 150–151
adenosine triphosphate
    (ATP) shortage, 102
adrenal depletion, 274–275
alcohol, avoiding of, 116, 200
Alexander Technique, 36
alpha-EEG anomaly, 19
Americans with Disabilities
    Act (ADA), 235–237
analgesics, 135–136
anger, 208–209
anticonvulsants, 138
antidepressants, 33, 125,
    133–135, 139, 269–270
apnea, 20–21, 76, 111–112.
    See also sleep

B

benzodiazepines, 137, 140
biofeedback, 225–226
bruxism, 112–113

C

caffeine, avoiding of,
    98, 105, 110, 200
candida (yeast)
    hypersensitivity,
    130–131, 275–277
carpal tunnel syndrome, 128
cervical stenosis, 278–280
Chiari malformation, 278–280
children, 68, 253–255
chiropractics, 153–155
chronic fatigue immune
    deficiency syndrome

(CFIDS), 12–13,
    31–34, 98–102
chronic myofascial pain
    (CMP), 13, 34–37, 156
clinical trials, 282–284
cognitive-behavioral
    therapy (CBT), 230
complementary and alternative
    medicine (CAM), 149–166
sources of information
    about, 163–164
types of, 150–162
confusion (fibro fog),
    6, 22, 117–118, 195
coping methods,
    167–180, 259–268
activities of daily living
    and, 175–180
body mechanics and, 170–175
phases of adaptation to
    disease and, 167–170
positive thinking and,
    180, 199–200, 215–217,
    219–220, 262–263
cosmetics, pain and, 85
creams, topical, 138–139
Crohn's disease, 24
cytokines, 101

D

denial, 208
dental problems, 123–124
depression, 6–7, 22–23,
    97, 119–120, 182, 207
diagnosis, 3–4, 67–78.
    See also symptoms
diet

fatigue and, 97–98
interstitial cystitis and, 126
irritable bowel syndrome
    and, 125
medications and, 144
pain and, 91–92
sleep and, 115–116
stress and, 196–197, 200–201
tips for healthy, 164–166
disability benefits, 240–243
dizziness, 132
doctors, see medical team

E

emotions, 10, 207–220
coping with, 212–220, 264–265
fatigue and, 106
typical of fibro patients,
    207–212
see also mind-body
    connection; stress
endocrinologist, 55
endometriosis, 40
endorphins, 87
Epstein-Barr virus, 12, 47
exercise, 92, 181–191,
    201, 261–262
types of, 184–188
eyes, dryness of, 122–123

F

family practice
    physician, 52–53
fatigue, 72, 95–106
factors contributing to, 97–102
managing of, 102–106
as symptom, 6, 21–22
see also chronic fatigue
    immune deficiency
    syndrome
fear, 210–211

fibro fog, 6, 22, 117–118, 195
fibromyalgia, 70, 72, 78
about, 1–9
conditions associated
    with or imitative of,
    12–15, 31–47, 71–72
future treatments for, 269–284
risk factors for, 8–9
suspected causes of, 9–11
see also diagnosis; symptoms
friendships, 255–256, 265–267

G

gastroesophageal reflux
    disease (GERD), 109
guaifenesin, 280
guided imagery, 226–227
guilt, 210
Gulf War veterans, 10

H

headaches, 25–27, 120–122, 141
heartburn, 109
herbal supplements, 158–162
list of, 160–162
hormones, 10–11, 88
hypersensitivity, 5, 129–131
hypnosis, 223–225
hypothalamic-pituitary-
    adrenal (HPA) axis, 11
hypothyroidism, 43–44,
    101–102, 276

I

idiopathic environmental
    intolerances (IEI), 129–130
imitators, of fibromyalgia,
    31–47, 71–72
infections, 10, 280–281
injections, 139

injuries, as suspected
  cause, 8, 9
insomnia, see sleep
internist, 53
interstitial cystitis, 24, 126, 141
irritable bowel syndrome
  (IBS), 23–24, 124–125, 141

L

leg movements, involuntary,
  20, 111, 137, 141
loneliness, 211–212
lupus, 13–14, 38–40
Lyme disease, 14–15, 40–43

M

marriage, 248–253
massage, 155–157
medical team, 49–65
choosing doctor, 59–63
kinds of practitioners, 50–59
your relationship with,
  49–50, 63–65, 261
medications, 133–147
antidepressants, 33, 125,
  133–135, 139, 269–270
cautions about, 139–
  140, 142–147
fatigue and, 98, 102–103
for headaches, 121–122
irritable bowel syndrome
  and, 125
keeping record of, 64
libido and, 251
over-the-counter, 58, 140, 146
for pain relief, 133–139
research on, 269–273
sleep and, 140–141
meditation, 222–223
menstrual problems, 25, 126

milnacipran, 269–270
mind-body connection,
  221–232
Mirapex, 272–273
mononucleosis, 47
mouth, dryness of, 122–123
multiple sclerosis (MS), 47
muscle pain, 13, 137–138, 229
myofascial pain, 13, 34–37, 156

N

nervous system, 9, 100–101
neurologist, 55–56
nicotine, 116
numbness, 128–129

O

obstetrician-gynecologist,
  54–55
occupational therapist, 57, 103
osteoarthritis, 46
osteopathic physician, 53–54

P

pain, 79–94
causes of, 85–94
exercise and, 189–190
gate control theory of, 88–89
medical relief from, 133–139
nervous system and, 80–84
normal versus fibro, 84–85
stress and, 195
as symptom, 5, 17–18
pain management specialist, 56
pediatrician, 55
periodic leg movements during
  sleep (PLMS), 20, 111
peripheral thyroid
  resistance, 277–278
pharmacist, 58

physiatrist, 56
physical therapist, 56–57, 103
placebo effect, 232
polymyalgia rheumatica, 47
positive thinking, 180, 199–200,
    215–217, 219–220, 262–263
posture, 172–173
prayer, 227–229
psychiatrist, 56
psychologist, 59
pyridostigmine, 270–271

Q

qi gong, 186–187

R

Raynaud's phenomenon,
    28, 132
Reiki, 157–158
relationships, 247–258
friendships, 255–256, 265–267
marriage, 248–253
parenthood, 253–255
support groups, 256–258
restless leg syndrome
    (RLS), 20, 110, 137, 141
rheumatoid arthritis, 14, 44–46
rheumatologist, 52

S

serotonin, 11, 87, 269–270
sleep, 103, 105–116
best positions for, 173–175
disturbances of, 11,
    18–21, 108–111
exercise and, 182
hormones and, 88
medications and, 140–141
pain and, 94
stages of normal, 107–108

stress and, 195, 198
ways to improve, 114–116
see also fatigue
Social Security Disability
    Insurance, 240–243
social worker, 59
stimulants, 140–141
stress, 92–94, 193–206
control of, 197–206, 263–264
substance P, 11, 67,
    76, 87, 113, 276
suicide, 23
support groups, 256–258
symptoms, 5–8, 17–29, 117–
    132. See also diagnosis

T

tai chi, 186
temporomandibular
    joint disorder (TMJ),
    27–28, 112, 123
testing, for fibromyalgia, 75–77
tingling, 128–129
topical creams, 138–139
travel, 244–246
trigger points, 18,
    35–36, 151–153

V

vulvodynia, 25, 127

W

walking, 188
water, 200, 245
work issues, 233–243

X

Xyrem, 271–272

Y

yoga, 185–186

The Everything® Health Guide Series

Supportive advice. Real answers.

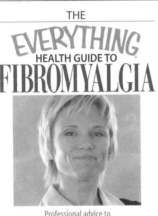

Trade Paperback
ISBN: 1-59337-586-7
$14.95 ($19.95 CAN)

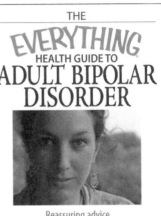

Trade Paperback
ISBN: 1-59337-585-9
$14.95 ($19.95 CAN)

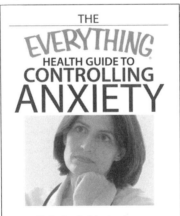

Trade Paperback
ISBN: 1-59337-429-1
$14.95 ($19.95 CAN)

Everything® and everything.com® are registered trademarks of F+W Publications, Inc.
Available wherever books are sold.
Or call us at 1-800-289-0963 or visit www.adamsmedia.com.